CW00552997

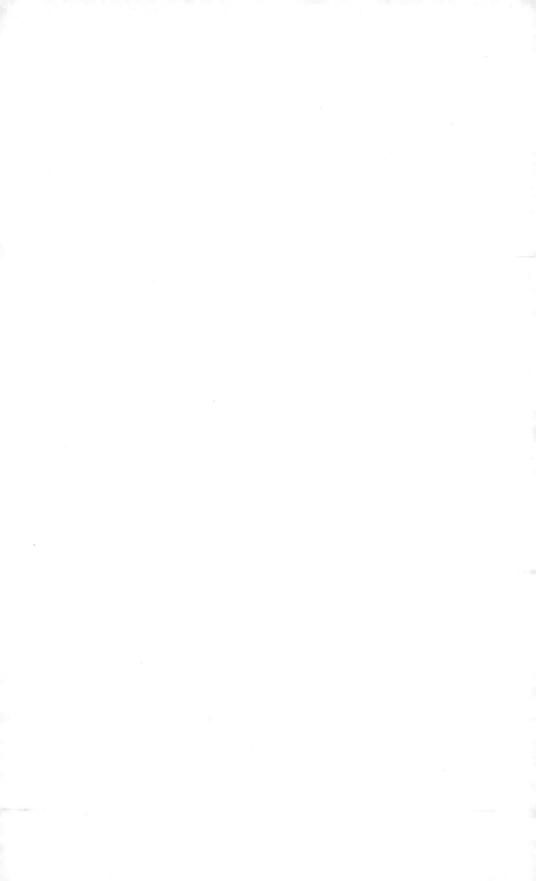

Deinstitutionalization and Community Living

Deinstitutionalization and Community Living

Intellectual disability services in Britain, Scandinavia and the USA

Edited by

Jim Mansell
University of Kent at Canterbury, UK

and

Kent Ericsson
University of Uppsala, Sweden

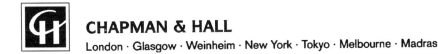

CHAPMAN & HALL
London · Glasgow · Weinheim · New York · Tokyo · Melbourne · Madras

Published by Chapman & Hall, 2–6 Boundary Row, London SE1 8HN, UK

Chapman & Hall, 2–6 Boundary Row, London SE1 8HN, UK

Blackie Academic & Professional, Wester Cleddens Road, Bishopbriggs, Glasgow G64 2NZ, UK

Chapman & Hall GmbH, Pappelallee 3, 69469 Weinheim, Germany

Chapman & Hall USA, 115 Fifth Avenue, New York NY 10003, USA

Chapman & Hall Japan, ITP-Japan, Kyowa Building, 3F, 2-2-1 Hirakawacho, Chiyoda-ku, Tokyo 102, Japan

Chapman & Hall Australia, 102 Dodds Street, South Melbourne, Victoria 3205, Australia

Chapman & Hall India, R. Seshadri, 32 Second Main Road, CIT East, Madras 600 035, India

Distributed in the USA and Canada by Singular Publishing Group Inc., 4284 41st Street, San Diego, California 92105

First edition 1996

© 1996 Chapman & Hall

Typeset in Palatino 10/12pt by Saxon Graphics Ltd, Derby
Printed in Great Britain

ISBN 0 412 57010 6   1 56593 315 X (USA)

A catalogue record for this book is available from the British Library.

∞ Printed on permanent acid-free text paper, manufactured in accordance with ANSI/NISO Z39.48-1992 and ANSI/NISO Z39.48-1984 (Permanence of Paper).

Contents

Contributors

Mary Ann Allard PhD
Centre for Social Policy Research
McCormack Institute
University of Massachusetts
at Boston
MA
USA

Valerie Bradley
President
Human Services Research Institute
MA
USA

Hilary Brown PhD
Senior Lecturer in Learning
Disability
Tizard Centre
University of Kent at Canterbury
Kent
UK

Paul Castellani PhD
Director of Programme Research
New York State Office of Mental
Retardation and Developmental
Disabilities
NY
USA

James Conroy PhD
Conroy Output Analysts, Inc.
PA
USA

Eric Emerson
Deputy Director
Hester Adrian Research Centre
University of Manchester
Manchester
UK

Kent Ericsson
Research Psychologist
Department of Education
Uppsala University
Uppsala
Sweden

Professor David Felce PhD
Director
Welsh Centre for Learning
Disabilities
Cardiff
UK

Chris Hatton
Research Fellow
Hester Adrian Research Centre
University of Manchester
Manchester
UK

Professor Jim Mansell
Director
Tizard Centre
University of Kent at Canterbury
Kent
UK

Danuta Orlowska
Lecturer in Learning Disability
Tizard Centre
University of Kent at Canterbury
Kent
UK

Timo Saloviita
University of Jyväskylä
Department of Special Education
Jyväskylä
Finland

Johans Sandvin
Nordlandsforskning
Mörkved
Bodö
Norway

Donald Shumway
Director
New Hampshire Division of
Mental Health
and Developmental Services
NH
USA

Barbro Tuvesson
Social Worker
Skövde
Sweden

Jan Tøssebro
Department of Sociology
University of Trondheim
Dragvoll
Norway

Foreword

Valerie Bradley
Vice-Chair and Presiding Officer of the US President's Committee on
Mental Retardation

The true consequences of major changes in any sphere of public policy are revealed in a frustratingly slow fashion. Even when dramatic shifts are accompanied by research on potential outcomes, there is no way of simulating the results of significant structural change, given the vagaries of execution and the inevitable slippage between aspirations and application. Ascertaining whether a particular course of action lives up to its promise is very difficult in the din and confusion of implementation. The shift in public policy that spurred the movement to close institutions and to place people with intellectual disabilities in homes in local communities is no exception.

While the reasons for deinstitutionalization are complex and vary across national political contexts, one common factor is the embrace by advocates of the concept of normalization and the rejection of segregation of people with intellectual disabilities from the rest of society. Institutions became both the symbol and the instrument of separation and the consequent stigmatization of people with intellectual disabilities. Reducing populations and ultimately closing institutions was the means by which residents could obtain the benefits accruing to all of living and participating in normal communities. The challenges presented by this goal were highly complex, in that the task entailed dismantling large bureaucratic structures on the one hand, and the creation of a new system of community resources on the other.

The 'first generation' of research in deinstitutionalization focused on the process of dismantling and charting the relocation outcomes for the people who were moved. Such studies were largely designed to answer the question: 'Are people better off in the community?' Studies also explored the political and administrative issues surrounding the closure of institutions including the impact of court intervention, the resistance of unionized institutional employees and the reactions of families to the placement of their relatives. This research proved useful in reassuring policy makers that institutional closures and phase-downs were not jeopardizing, but rather enhancing the well-being of those relocated, and pointed out important lessons for state and local administrators saddled with the task of hastening the decline of large public facilities. While this initial wave of research was important, its utility will continue to decline as more and more countries phase down large institutions over the next decade. In the United States, the institutional population has declined from a peak of 194 659 in 1967 (Lakin et al., 1989) to only about 75 000 in June 1992 (Gettings, 1992b), and several states including Rhode Island, Vermont and New Hampshire no longer maintain large public institutions for people with intellectual disabilities.

In other words, knowing how to close institutions for people with intellectual disabilities will eventually be equivalent to knowing how to treat polio – the job will ultimately be completed. Obviously, the decline in institutional populations is taking place at different rates in different countries given resource and political differences. Countries such as those in central Europe, where institutional populations are still significant, will continue to benefit from experience elsewhere. For the future, however, the more interesting questions will be those that focus on the second phase of reform – the development of a viable, stable, and high quality system of community resources. The question in this phase is not simply whether people are better off than they were in the community, but whether their lives provide the same opportunities for socialization and inclusion in their communities as for the rest of the population, with all the implications for individually-tailored support that that entails.

The analyses presented in this volume represent, in most instances, 'second generation' research on deinstitutionalization – that is, research that digs beneath the initial studies of closure and focuses on the variables within community programmes and in administrative support structures that are predictive of better outcomes – how do staff attitudes and their interaction with people with intellectual disabilities affect the progress of community residents? How can families be collaborators in planning and developing resources for their family members? What is the impact of increasing decentralization of authority and responsibility and the decline of specialized services to people with intellectual disabilities in favour of an integrated, 'dedifferentiated' local system of social services? The answers to these questions are important to the expansion of reform and to the design and enhancement of community systems of support.

Many of the authors in this book speak to the successes of the movement of people out of institutions including positive changes in the attitudes of families, positive changes in the individuals who left, and the expansion of community resources. However, it is clearly too early to declare victory – at least in the fight to establish high quality community services – given some of the warning flags also raised by the findings that follow. As the headlines of success in early skirmishes to downsize institutions has subsided, more sobering and equally complex issues have arisen that may threaten continued progress and that should cause a reassessment of the limited goal of dismantling and relocation. Some of these issues include structural and training issues surrounding the conduct of community services, changes in the political and economic climate, potential loss of entitlements and rights in a decentralized generic social services system, and a reduction of those welfare state benefits that make it possible to maintain people in communities and to keep them out of institutions in the first place.

Looking beyond successful relocation, we are now able to discern differences in the quality of the community programmes established over the past two decades. From the vantage point of the 1990s, we can see that many community programmes, while providing better care and physical surroundings for people with intellectual disabilities, did not provide a social and psychological milieu that was materially different than that in the remote, segregated institutions that preceded them. This closer examination of the content rather than the form of community services has generated an interest in the quality of life of individual residents, as reflected in their participation in communities and the extent to which they are participants in the choices that affect their lives.

A NEW PARADIGM OF COMMUNITY SERVICES

The recognition that deinstitutionalization should be more than just 'a change of address' coincides with the emergence of a 'new paradigm' or set of assumptions regarding the conduct of services to people with intellectual disabilities. This new set of assumptions acknowledges that people with intellectual disabilities are capable of making choices about their own lives, respects their right to do so, and focuses on individualized supports and empowerment. Bradley and Knoll (1995) identify four major attributes of this new paradigm, primacy of community, emphasis on relationships, person-centred supports, and choice and control. These revised priorities have a profound impact on how services are provided:

- The primacy of the community – The new paradigm rests on the fundamental belief that people with disabilities can and should live in communities as full participating members. The role of service providers is to identify and remove barriers to full community participation.

- Emphasis on relationships – People with disabilities have the same needs for social connectedness as do any other persons living in communities. A fundamental task of service providers is to ensure that people make social connections and become fully integrated into the life of the community. These social relationships make it possible for people with disabilities to make use of natural supports in their communities.
- Person-centred supports – This view of services for people with disabilities eschews the notion of fitting people into available programme 'slots'. Rather supports must be designed to respond to the unique situation of each individual in his or her community. People with disabilities should live in homes, not in programmes and they should work in jobs, not in workshops. Programme planning must include the full array of family members, friends, service providers, advocates and, most importantly, the consumer.
- Choice and control – The new paradigm rejects the notion that 'the professionals know best'. Instead, it recognizes the right of consumers to make choices about where and with whom they live, how they spend their time and how they want their supports configured. The task for community support workers is to assist consumers in making informed choices and to ensure that meaningful choices are available.

IMPLICATIONS FOR STAFF

A focus on quality of life and community membership requires a reconfiguration of staffing patterns and staff training. Services are increasingly being delivered in homes, workplaces, schools and communities, and are therefore more and more decentralized. The nature of the work is also changing. The role of direct care staff in traditional organizations is essentially to be the arms and legs of the agency, carrying out orders rather than collaborating to solve problems. Though direct service personnel are often asked to work in highly decentralized and isolated circumstances, they are rarely given the autonomy to shape their work life. In more individualized settings, they will likely be called on to make independent decisions, to work with people with intellectual disabilities and their families to fashion individual and idiosyncratic supports, and to work with generic agencies and natural supports in unique and community specific configurations.

Dramatic increases in the numbers and types of community-based support settings have mixed implications for staff: greater autonomy and responsibility may increase commitment and job satisfaction but make recruitment, retention and training more difficult (Larson, Hewitt and Lakin, 1994). Multiple settings also increase the probability of poor fit between the expectations of new recruits and the job requirements resulting in higher turnover (Ebenstein and Gooler, 1993). Scheduling and arranging for training is more difficult across multiple settings (Langer, Agosta and Choisser, 1988).

Mittler (1987), in commenting on staff development needs in Great Britain, made the following observation:

> There is a sense in which we are all unqualified and ill prepared even to meet today's needs. The speed and scale of change, even within the last ten years, the flood of new information on changing practice, are so great that much of what is taught to new staff is becoming dated even before they complete their training. How much greater, then, is the challenge of helping existing staff to modify their practice and attitudes in the light of the changes that have taken place since they started working in this field? How, too, do we create an awareness of the needs of people with disabilities in the countless numbers of staff working in ordinary services?
>
> (Mittler, 1987, p.31)

This changing vision of how services should be delivered to people with intellectual disabilities has major implications for the types of workers required and the training these workers need. As Knoll and Racino (1994) note:

> The basic values of personal choice and control, individual quality of life, valued roles, and full community participation for people with developmental disabilities does indeed require the fundamental transformation of words and practice inherent in the support paradigm. However, this promise will be lost if the field does not systematically reeducate itself and develop new workers who are both imbued in this new way of thinking and have the skills needed to undertake the far reaching changes that lie ahead.
>
> (Knoll and Racino, 1994, p.5)

Community staff will need to be taught skills that are qualitatively different from those geared to more structured settings. Some of these qualities have been identified by the Family Empowerment Project at Cornell University for people engaged in generic family support:

- Ability and commitment to identifying strengths in people and groups;
- Genuine respect for diverse perspectives and life styles;
- A capacity to listen and reflect;
- An ability to subordinate one's own ego (to put one's self aside in the interest of the group);

- Skill and creativity in helping people become more aware and confident of their own abilities;
- Appreciation of when to step back and the ability to help the individual or group assume decision-making and action;
- Ability to analyse power relationships and help others to do so;
- Knowledge about how to gain access to information;
- Ability to reflect on and criticise ongoing process, including one's own role in those processes.

(Cochran, 1990)

POLITICAL AND ECONOMIC IMPLICATIONS

A further challenge, noted by many of the authors in this volume, is the rapidly changing political and economic climate in the United States and Western Europe. We are reminded that the era of deinstitutionalization and community expansion occurred during a period of expanding resources and optimism. The motivation for reform was primarily to further ideological ends such as normalization, and to implement what was determined to be a rational policy (e.g. based on cost comparisons, research findings, quality issues, etc.). However, the current landscape is dramatically altered. Instead of expanding resources the challenge today is to do more with less. Instead of an expanding welfare state, national governments are developing plans to circumscribe benefits and services. Instead of centralized authority and vision, the catchphrase is devolution, local control and block grants.

Thus, the next wave of reform – building community capacity – is occurring in a period of constriction and political retrenchment. Progressive ideology has shifted to fiscal conservatism and the motives that guided deinstitutionalization may be turned to a more cynical attempt to shift responsibility and avoid more expensive specialized services. The lowered expectations generated by the emerging political mood has significant ramifications for both the quality of community services as well as the availability of services and supports to those at home with their families.

Growth in the numbers of people with intellectual disabilities receiving publicly-supported services in the United States has been reasonably slow, increasing by an average of only ½% per year since 1967 (Gettings, 1992b). Thus, the beneficiaries of the rapid expansion of services in the 1970s and 1980s were those individuals who were moved out of institutions, and the aspirations of thousands of people with intellectual disabilities were effectively placed 'on hold'. In a 1987 publication by the Association for Retarded Citizens of the United States, the number of individuals with mental retardation on waiting lists for community services nationwide was 132 967. By 1991, the University of Minnesota estimated that this figure had grown to 196 000. Given the continuing revenue shortfalls in many states around the United States, it is reasonable to assume that this is now a conservative figure.

Further, it is becoming clear that the political commitment needed to sustain the continued expansion of the highly specialized and increasingly expensive models of residential and day services developed during the 1970s and early 1980s cannot be relied upon. Gettings (1992) has estimated that to meet the residential demand in the United States, states would have to increase their residential budgets by a full 20%. In reflecting on the fiscal realities at the federal and state level, Gettings makes the following observation:

> The resources are simply not available – and not likely to be available in the foreseeable future – to sustain the growth rate in spending which the field experienced during the past decade. Further expansions and improvements in services to people with developmental disabilities, therefore will be largely dependent on the capacity of advocates, providers and state officials to join hands in charting a new course that emphasises more efficient utilisation of available human and fiscal resources.
>
> (Gettings, 1992b, p.16)

The fiscal and political context also poses challenges to the continued quality of those community programmes that exist. To the extent that quality is compromised, the covenant that we have made with families regarding the safety and well-being of their family members in the community may be jeopardized. A lack of trust on the part of families coupled with the perceived 'economies of scale' inherent in congregate settings could result in an erosion of the momentum to create individualized supports for people with intellectual disabilities. Continued collaboration with family members and people with intellectual disabilities as well as professionals will be needed to maintain the gains made in the past two decades and to expand services and supports to those individuals who have never been institutionalized.

CHANGES IN THE WELFARE STATE

Another important issue described in this volume is the overlay of decentralization initiatives and deinstitutionalization. In some countries, the move to decentralize, though occurring contemporaneously, was not directly linked to deinstitutionalization. In Norway, the two initiatives were expressly linked. Decentralization and devolution of authority to counties and municipalities in much of Western Europe has resulted in the integration of services to people with intellectual disabilities into generic social services programmes. Decentralization is also taking place in the United States and while most services to people with intellectual disabilities remain separate, consolidation of health related services under the rubric of 'managed care' may also result in the loss of a categorical identity for such services.

On one level, removing the 'special' character of services to people with intellectual disabilities can be seen as the next step toward normalization. On the other hand, such dedifferentiation, as Sandvin has characterized it, can also result in a loss of special entitlements and the specialized expertise necessary to respond to the complex challenges of people with severe and profound intellectual disabilities. Decentralization and dedifferentiation also mean that decisions about resources must be made among competing local priorities including those of the elderly, children, people with physical handicaps, drug abusers, as well as people with intellectual disabilities. This means that conventional advocacy organizations that have by and large functioned at the national level will have to organize locally and will have to build thoughtful alliances with other constituencies.

Anders Gustavsson, from the Stockholm College of Health and Caring Sciences, also addressed some of these tensions in a speech at the 11th Annual Young Adult Institute Conference in New York City. In commenting on the decentralization phenomenon, Gustavsson (1990) noted a potentially ironic consequence:

> There might be a growing risk that persons with severe handicaps in Sweden, as those who can't handle the service system effectively, in the future may not be in a position to benefit from the services provided. The paradoxical situation may occur, where the quality of life improves considerably for the competent and strong persons, while the remainder get worse conditions than before as a result of the very same development. This brings us back to the question of quality and equality of life, which may be one of the most important future issues in integrated society.
>
> (Gustavsson, 1990, p.7)

IMPACT OF REDUCED ENTITLEMENTS

A final issue that should be of increasing concern as we attempt to solidify gains made in community services and take the next step to enhance and expand community support is the possibility of a diminishing safety net for people with intellectual disabilities. In the United States, there are currently discussions at the federal level that may result in a significant decrease in pensions for families who have children with intellectual disabilities, in vocational services, in federally supported health care, and in maternal and child health services. These same conversations are also taking place in many other countries. Clearly, by diminishing income and other financial supports, it will be difficult for families to maintain family members with intellectual disabilities in the community and to support adults in their own homes and on the job. Ironically, the very entitlements that made it possible for people to find alternatives to institutionalization may be diminished to a level that pressure for institutionalization will once again increase – not because people prefer this option, but because their desperation may lead them to this 'Hobson's choice'.

CONCLUSION

The chapters that follow are testimony to the massive strides that have been made in the reform of services to people with intellectual disabilities through the phasing down of institutions and the creation of community alternatives. No one who has been involved in this process can be in any doubt that it is possible, given imagination, skills and resources, to greatly improve the lives of people with intellectual disabilities as members of the societies in which they live. In by far the majority of cases, the dismantling of institutions has resulted in lives for former residents that are better than those they lived in large public facilities. This success rests not upon a simplistic or naïve view of what needs to be done, but upon hard-won understanding of the problems and pitfalls that have to be faced to do the job properly.

It is recognized, though, that the success of the replacement of institutions and the development of community capacity is still elusive. It is contingent on our ability to recruit and train support staff, to maximize public as well as family and community supports, to ensure adequate advocacy for people with intellectual disabilities in decentralized settings, and to persuade local and national policy makers that any reduction of financial supports is a false economy that may ultimately result in reinstitutionalization and resegregation. Safeguarding the future therefore means, for all of us, not only finding better ways of meeting the needs and aspirations of people with intellectual disabilities, but also engaging with the wider political debate about equality of opportunity and civil rights.

Preface

The chapters of this book were originally presented as papers at a symposium at the Centre for Handicap Research at Uppsala University. The symposium was made possible through grants from the Swedish Council for Social Research, the Sävstaholm Foundation and the Skinfaxe Institute, to whom thanks are due.

Contributors to this volume have used different terms to refer to people using the services under examination. In Scandinavian countries the term used in English is 'mental retardation'; in the United States this term is used alongside 'developmental disabilities', which usually includes a slightly wider definition. In Britain, the term 'mental handicap' has been replaced in official use by the term 'learning disabilities'; the phrase 'learning difficulties' is also in widespread use. In international use the term 'intellectual disabilities' has found favour.

Since there are marginal differences in these definitions, we have followed the editorial practice of retaining the usage of each author rather than converting them all to one common phrase. In the first and last chapters, and in the introduction to each section of the book, we have used the term 'intellectual disabilities'.

The editors would like to thank Kathy Bugden of the Tizard Centre for her help in preparing the manuscript for publication.

Jim Mansell, Canterbury, Kent
Kent Ericsson, Uppsala, Sweden
May 1995

Introduction: towards deinstitutionalization

1

Kent Ericsson and Jim Mansell

Deinstitutionalization has been perhaps the most important development in the way services for people with intellectual disabilities have been organized in Western Europe and North America over the last 25 years. The book *Changing patterns in Residential Services for the Mentally Retarded* (Kugel and Wolfensberger, 1969) represented a turning point in thinking about services, summarizing the shift from traditional forms of institutional care of the 1950s and 1960s to new models based on the community, and elaborating new objectives and ideals for the change towards community services.

The following ten years was a period when community services were first being established. Ideas and models were formulated and tried out. Although at first offered primarily to people with mild or moderate intellectual disabilities, community services came to be so well developed that they could even offer support to those with the most extensive needs. They became, therefore, attractive alternatives even for people who were living in institutions. With the growth of community services new ideals also developed. The conditions and quality of life which could thus be offered began to be seen as the standard, against which the large institutions were to be judged.

These were also the years during which work was carried out to change the large institutions. Extensive programmes of refurbishment and development were often attempted. But increasingly, in a situation where those responsible were faced with the choice of reforming institutions or allowing the residents to move to community forms of service, many chose the latter alternative. As sufficient numbers of people left, the institutions could be closed down. During the later part of the 1970s the process of closure of institutions began in Sweden, as it did in the United States and Britain. The 1980s came to be the decade when this task began to be realized on any scale, as the development of community services reached sufficient levels to permit the final abandonment of institutional care.

Now it is possible to look forward to the end of the traditional institution in the care of people with intellectual disabilities. The major questions about services no longer concern the feasibility of replacing institutions but the nature of replacement services and the extent to which these societies are politically committed to enabling people with intellectual disabilities to realize their potential as citizens.

From a perspective which focuses on the person during the process of change, there are dramatic changes in the circumstances under which people live and in their quality of life. In general, community services are quite different from the institutions they replace in the material richness of the living environment, the opportunity they provide for greater privacy, choice and independence and in the scale and quality of the relationships they offer. When people move they can experience important and multifaceted improvements in their conditions, discovering new ways of living, new activities and new relationships within the ordinary community.

Traditionally, those adults with extensive need for support have been referred to institutional care, a life outside the institution being first and foremost provided for those with less extensive needs. When community services first began to be offered to those previously offered institutional care, a long tradition was broken. It required extensive development in order to establish community services which could meet the requirements of those with extensive needs. In particular, this meant distinguishing between the living conditions or opportunities presented by new services in the community and the organization and effectiveness of support to the people served to enable them to live a rich and full life. In this process of service development a foundation was laid for the future organization of services and support to be provided by society.

As the people involved will be greatly affected by this change, and the services created will form a basis for future developments, there is good reason to analyse the process which is taking place. The purpose of this book is to take stock, in the middle of the 1990s, of progress in deinstitutionalization, drawing on the experience of the countries of Scandinavia, the United States and Britain. There is now a relatively large store of experience and evidence about the closure of institutions, the development of community services and the effects of deinstitutionalization on people with intellectual disabilities and their families. Contributors have therefore been able both to describe relevant work in the field and reflect on it to identify the lessons that can be learned and the issues which remain to be addressed.

This book takes as its starting point the declining numbers of people with intellectual disabilities in institutions. Much has already been written about the origins of institutional care (Wolfensberger, 1975; Rothman, 1971; Foucault, 1967; Scull, 1993) and the way in which institutions developed. The reader is referred to these sources for this background material. It is, however, interesting to note that institutions for people with intellectual disabilities began as a humane response to the oppression and misery of the general workhouse, and the lack of support in increasingly industrialized communities. They became perverted by the influence of eugenicist ideas and the unremitting pressure for more places from communities where exclusion was offered as the preferred alternative. The deinstitutionalization movement has its origins in the Second World War – which focused attention on the problems of social adjustment and dislocation among refugees and displaced persons, i.e. women and children evacuated from cities under air attack and, above all, on trying to understand the concentration camps – and led to a critical re-evaluation of institutional care and social exclusion. Alternatives to institutional care were pioneered for increasing numbers of disabled people and when policy and social conditions in the 1960s favoured a change in practice it was possible to begin the gradual abandonment of institutional care.

AN OVERVIEW OF DEINSTITUTIONALIZATION IN SCANDINAVIA, THE UNITED STATES AND BRITAIN

Figure 1.1 shows the decline in the number of places in institutions for people with intellectual disabilities in Sweden, Norway, the United States, England and Wales over the last 25 years. The numbers have been converted to rates per 100 000 total population in order to permit comparisons. These data are drawn from different sources* and there are some minor inconsistencies between, and discontinuities within, the national series, but the overall trends and levels illustrate the nature of the changes which have taken place.

*English and Welsh data from *Health and Personal Social Services Statistics for England and Health and Personal Social Services Statistics for Wales*; Swedish data from the National Board of Welfare and National Statistics Office; Norwegian data from Tøssebro (personal communication); American data from Braddock *et al.* (1995) and Scheerenberger (1981); Population data from *United Nations Monthly Bulletin of Statistics* and (for England and Wales) from *Office of Population Censuses and Surveys Population Trends*.

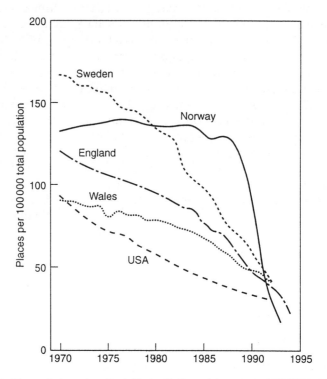

Figure 1.1 Places in learning disability institutions (places per 100 000 total population).

In the United States the picture is of steady substantial decline over the whole period, becoming slightly less steep in later years. In Sweden, England and Wales the decline during the 1970s increases during the 1980s and 1990s. In Norway the onset of deinstitutionalization is much later, although as Tøssebro points out in Chapter 5, this is in part artefactual since many of the institutions are small and would be called group homes in other countries. The variation in institutional provision across different countries must be interpreted with caution, since they may to some extent reflect a different balance between types of service rather than different overall levels of provision of residential care. Nevertheless, it is plausible that Sweden and Norway, with a long tradition of investment in public services, should provide most services, and that England and Wales, providing institutional care through a National Health Service, should also provide more than the United States, with its commitment to free enterprise and cautious approach to public services.

SCANDINAVIA

The entire post-war period in Sweden has been characterized by a process of change, with the development of community services and the move away from institutional care. It has primarily been concerned with children and young people, and people with mild intellectual disability. Consequently, boarding schools and children's homes have gradually disappeared. These developments, however, affected adults with extensive need for support much later (Ericsson, 1985b) and it is only now that community services are being developed to replace the remaining institutions.

In Norway it was not until after the Second World War that particular interest was shown in these services. A period of extensive building was initiated after 1949 with legislation on the development of institutional services, to be financed with state funds. This process continued until 1976, since when the number of places in institutions have not increased. Towards the end of the 1960s a period of institutional improvement began, concentrating on developing the services within these institutions. This period was characterized by an ambition to reduce the size of institutions, introduce a greater degree of decentralization, make the wards more home-like and develop their educational and occupational facilities. These suggested improvements were a response to criticism of institutions and the demands which originated in the normalization principle. The beginning of the 1990s has seen the start of a period of closure, furthered by the law which states that special county services for persons with intellectual disabilities should be discontinued from 1992 (Tøssebro, 1992).

The dissolution of institutions has also become a reality in Finland where from 1977 government has supported the shift towards community services, breaking a trend which had existed since the 1940s and which had led to an increased number of places in institutions. This trend has changed and institutional closure has begun (Saloviita, 1990).

In Iceland early forms of services were institutional. Attitudes to these changed in the middle of the 1970s when emphasis began to be placed on the importance of parents being able to keep their children at home while they were growing up and, as adults, being able to live in the local community, in housing with adequate support. Today, a debate is taking place about the role of institutions (Thorarinsson, 1987) at the same time as the process of dissolution has begun. In Denmark services for persons with intellectual disabilities have always been dominated by large institutions, though changes have taken place to reduce their size. Work has also begun on the dissolution of some of them, with one already having been closed (Salomonsen, 1988).

The academic literature in Scandinavia starts with a critique of institutional care at the beginning of the 1970s. In the late 1970s and the early 1980s much attention was given to institutional reform, but since the mid-1980s the emphasis has shifted to institutional replacement.

Rasmussen (1972) offered a critique of institutions inspired by ideas of normalization, integration and democratization, views which were relatively new within this field. During the same period criticism of institutions can also to be found in Kylén's (1972) article 'An analysis of objectives for residential services' where, using the specified requirements on housing for persons with intellectual handicaps, he rejected the Swedish special hospitals as unacceptable places for the provision of care.

An early report of the development and improvement of existing facilities was Hansen's (1978) paper which discussed the question 'Can large institutions be detotalized?' Abrahamsson and Söder (1979) discussed forms of development of the internal organization of work in an institution in their article 'Changing institutions'. Lindman (1982) also accounted for a project on the development of institutions in the article 'The internal workings of an institution'. A project on working methods used on wards in residential institutions was reported by Kaipio (1983) in the article 'Pedagogics in the institution'.

A series of articles, all published during the 1980s or later, which concerned deinstitutionalization, started with a report from a Scandinavian symposium on 'The independence of wards' (Dam et al., 1982). A conclusion drawn at this symposium was that developments within institutions must be part of a process of which the final objective is to leave the institution in order to 'establish small local housing in the ordinary community. For all.' (Engberg, 1982). Later articles have dealt with various questions concerning, for example, the preparation of a plan for closure of an institution (Ericsson et al., 1983) and the tasks surrounding different issues involved in the closure of an institution (Brusén and Lerman, 1986). Sociopolitical aspects and economic consequences in connection with the closure of large institutions were discussed by Nielsen (1983) and Schultz (1984).

Fasting (1987) gives an account of the work which has been carried out on the closure of institutions in Norway. In Iceland the shift away from institutions has led to the decision being made to close one of the five institutions in the country (Thorsteinsdóttir and Björnsdottir, 1991).

That the closure of institutions is also concerned with the development of alternatives has been pointed out by Ericsson et al. (1980), Sonn (1984), Grunewald (1987) and Brusén (1990). Schmidt (1985) and Dam (1985) have pointed out that the task is not just to leave the old physical structures which institutions are made of, but to discard completely the way of thinking and the institutional culture which they represent.

Perlt (1990) summarizes the attitudes towards residential institutions in three phases. The first refers to the work carried out to bring the institutions into being, the second to change their content from a medical emphasis to a more social and pedagogical system of care, and the third phase concerns the task of opposing these institutions in order to achieve their closure and encourage the establishment of external services.

Thus, the overall picture is that the 1970s primarily involved projects which aimed at the development of institutional services, whereas the 1980s was the decade when their dissolution began. Hautamäki (1987) points out that this has been a process which has affected everyone involved in services for persons with intellectual handicaps and that the dissolution of institutions is recognized as a task of fundamental socio-political importance in Scandinavian societies.

UNITED STATES OF AMERICA

The provision of institutional care in the United States increased continuously from its establishment in the middle of the last century up until 1967, when the numbers first began to decrease. The peak was 194 650 people then receiving this form of care (Lakin *et al.*, 1981). The move towards community services has its origins in the 1950s when parents, through their criticism, turned their attention towards the conditions offered in institutions. During the 1960s, programmes to develop new forms of services were carried out and by the beginning of the 1970s these began to be implemented, emerging as the desirable way of providing services (Bruininks *et al.*, 1981).

The point at which the first formal renunciation of the institutional system of service took place was in 1963, when in a report President Kennedy pointed to the desirability of a decentralized community service. This was later underlined by President Nixon's pronouncement of the goal that one-third of those living in residential institutions should have left them before 1981. The 1970s can therefore be seen as the first decade of deinstitutionalization, leading to a reduction in the number of places in institutions (Bruininks *et al.*, 1981).

There were, however, more tangible events which gave impetus to the development away from institutional services. The foremost of these was Blatt and Rivera's publicity about the conditions inside institutions (Willer and Intagliata, 1984; Craig and McCarver, 1984). Litigation between representatives of people with intellectual disabilities and those running the services also contributed to this process. Scheerenberger (1981) dates the turning point for the commencement of deinstitutionalization to 1972, the year of the Wyatt v. Stickney case, which led to a ruling that persons with a mild form of intellectual disability should not be admitted to a residential institution.

The idea of normalization (Wolfensberger, 1972) also contributed to the move away from institutions (Craig and McCarver, 1984). Willer and Intagliata (1984) and Latib *et al.* (1984) suggest that the reaction against institutional services, as well as the move towards normalization, can also be found in the two expressions 'the developmental model' (Wolfensberger, 1969) and 'the least restrictive environment' (Turnbull *et al.*, 1981).

As in Scandinavia, deinstitutionalization for people with intellectual disabilities was at first coupled with aspirations for institutional renovation. Kugel said that institutions for persons with intellectual handicaps were a 'disgrace to the nation' (Kugel and Wolfensberger, 1969). The life that people were compelled to live in institutions was, he maintained, similar to the life animals led in a zoo. He identified three problems: too many people living in the institutions, insufficient staff, and lack of financial resources to offer a good standard of care. Scheerenberger (1976) suggested that quality was lacking in institutional services because of staff deficiencies, both numerically and in terms of competence. Institutions also made it possible, because of their physical structure, to promote 'mass-living', i.e. life in large groups. They did not, therefore, provide any opportunity for maximum human development and, he maintained, it was the quality of institutional services which should be discussed rather than institutions as such.

Novak and Berkely (1984) point to societal circumstances in the United States which favoured the shift away from institutions and the development of new types of services. They claimed that the attention given in American society to the Second World War and the economic expansion of the 1950s, had taken away attention from social matters. These therefore became more acceptable subjects for criticism and discussion during the 1960s, when rights and reactions against the war in Vietnam had become big social and political issues. Development took place within the framework of 'the open society'; a society which had begun to discuss the living conditions of various groups of citizens (Willer and Intagliata, 1984). Braddock *et al.* (1995) have also highlighted the importance of the civil rights tradition in explaining the progress made by different states in replacing institutions. By 1994, Braddock *et al.*, report that there were 94 scheduled or completed institutional closures in 29 states.

BRITAIN

Alternatives to institutional care in Britain began to be seriously considered in the 1950s when the demand for residential care appeared to be steadily increasing. The Report of the Royal Commission on the Law Relating to Mental Illness and Mental Deficiency, 1954–57 (1957) recommended that more provision should be made for people with mild intellectual disabilities in residential homes ('hostels') in the community, partly in order to relieve pressure on hospital places. The responsibility for community services lay with local, rather than central, government and little was done until, in the mid-1960s, a series of public scandals in institutions revealed extensive ill-treatment and neglect in squalid, overcrowded surroundings (Report of the Committee of Inquiry at Farleigh Hospital, 1971; Report of the Committee of Inquiry on Normansfield Hospital, 1978; Report of the Committee of Inquiry into South Ockendon Hospital, 1974; Report of the Committee of Inquiry into Whittingham Hospital, 1972; Martin, 1984; Morris, 1969). In response to this a Government White Paper (Department of Health and Social Security, 1971) reinforced the goal of providing community services for people with mild or moderate intellectual disabilities, and set unusually clear targets for local authority services. This initiative applied to England and Wales: Scotland has a different legislative framework and, generally, has been much slower to develop community services (Emerson and Hatton, 1994).

Also at the beginning of the 1970s, a new lobby developed, focused on an organization called Campaign for the Mentally Handicapped, which for the first time called for the complete abandonment of hospital care and its replacement by housing-based services in the community (Campaign for the Mentally Handicapped, 1970; 1972). This lobby drew its inspiration partly from the first community services in the United States and Scandinavia, and partly from earlier British work by Tizard (1960; 1964) demonstrating the superiority of community-based services.

In the early part of the 1970s, most new developments in the community were of large (20–25 person) units (Felce, Kushlick and Mansell, 1980a; 1980b; Felce, Mansell and Kushlick, 1980a; 1980b; Heron and Phillips, 1977; Hemming et al., 1979; Hemming, Lavender and Pill, 1981; Hemming, 1982), including some for people with severe and profound intellectual disabilities. By the middle of the decade, however, there was increasing pressure for housing-based services for all and the first examples of supported housing for people with severe or profound intellectual disabilities appeared (Mansell, 1976; 1977; 1980; Design for Special Needs, 1977).

Policy in Wales and England diverged at this point. In Wales, criticism of institutional refurbishment at Ely – the first institution for people with intellectual disabilities to have a major scandal – led to a demonstration project to serve a whole sector of the city of Cardiff with community-based services (Cardiff and Vale of Glamorgan Community Health Councils, 1977; Welsh Office, 1978; Lowe and de Paiva, 1991). The shift in thinking this entailed was later reflected in a national policy (the 'All-Wales Strategy') of developing community-based services and (consequently) closing institutions. Revision of this policy after a decade (Welsh Office, 1991; 1992) showed substantial development of community services by local authorities using earmarked central government funds, though with little impact on institutional numbers. In the second decade closure was identified as a key priority, though recently there has been some evidence of the lessening of central government commitment due to the issue of community care being redefined as a local government responsibility.

In England, government policy did not really address the question of whether all people with intellectual disabilities should be supported in ordinary housing. The main policy initiative in the 1970s focused on transferring funds from the health service (responsible for institutions) to local government. By the beginning of the 1980s, another official committee (Report of the Committee of Enquiry into Mental Handicap Nursing and Care, 1979) recommended housing-based services as the main future model of care, the Department of Health funded a research and development project in Andover (Mansell *et al.*, 1987; Felce, 1989) and the influential King's Fund Centre (King's Fund, 1980) published a report outlining the elements of community services needed to provide 'An Ordinary Life'.

These initiatives were followed by a national demonstration project called the 'Care in the Community' initiative, which used central government funding to enable 11 schemes to give local agencies experience of collaborating in transferring people from institutional to community care (Cambridge *et al.*, 1994; Davies and Challis, 1986). Although the schemes themselves were not necessarily very radical, this programme was important both because it signalled central government's overall acceptance of the policy goal of deinstitutionalization and because it gave many local service agencies experience of the work involved. In the second half of the 1980s the first large-scale institutional closures took place, at Darenth Park in Kent (Korman and Glennerster, 1985; 1990) and Starcross in Devon (Radford and Tipper, 1988) and the process gathered momentum, with deinstitutionalization becoming tacitly accepted as a general policy goal.

Also in the mid-1980s, there were policy developments concerned primarily with services for old people and people with mental health problems which were eventually to have a major impact on intellectual disability. Official concern about the rapidly increasing number of old people entering residential care funded by social security (Report of the Joint Central and Local Government Working Party on Public Support for Retardation, 1987), and evidence (Davies and Challis, 1986) that there was considerable inefficiency (the most disabled old people struggling on at home while less dependent people entered residential care), led to several official and quasi-official reviews (Griffiths, 1988; Audit Commission, 1986; House of Commons Social Services Committee, 1985). From these came major legislative reform in the 1990 Health and Community Care Act. This began to close the social security funding route and to impose on local authorities the responsibility for funding residential care. In future hospital care was to be almost solely concerned with short-term treatment. A further innovation was the requirement that most residential services purchased by local authorities were in future to be run by private-sector or voluntary organizations.

New guidance on intellectual disability, issued in 1992 (Department of Health, 1992; NHS Management Executive, 1992) again emphasized non-institutional services but, in a way characteristic of English policy-making in this field, stated that a range of service models (including larger, congregate settings) continued to be acceptable. The choice, however, of small-scale community-based models or institutional care continues to depend largely on decision-makers in health and local authorities rather than on any national legislative or policy commitment.

STRUCTURE OF THE BOOK

It is an understatement to say that deinstitutionalization is a complex process of change. When the institutional tradition, established more than 100 years ago, is faced with alternative forms of support and service which eventually will lead to the closure of institutions, many new tasks will, of course, arise, both in the development of new services and the dissolution of the old.

The complexity of this process of change is increased as it is not only a question of finding ways of providing support and services to people with intellectual disabilities. Residential institutions have also developed into large places of employment and when they are reduced in size, or totally closed down, the change also involves the issue of employment and the need for alternatives for staff. In the areas where these institutions have been located they have often played an important economic role in the local community, a factor which contributes to the many interests having to be taken into consideration during the task of deinstitutionalization.

In the production of alternatives to institutions lies the creative task, not only of building new placements in the community but also of avoiding reproduction of the same type of care which was available at the institution. Instead, community services require new ways of organizing services and providing help and support to people with intellectual disabilities, especially for those with the most extensive needs. Institutional populations include people with widely varying needs and aspirations and the development of good services requires highly individualized planning and service delivery. In some ways the concept of deinstitutionalization focuses on the institution and thereby emphasizes an organizational perspective. Community services require that attention is focused instead at the personal level, concentrating on the person, in need of support and services, as the nucleus for the process of change.

These themes – closure and development, organization and individual – are reflected in the chapters which follow. The book is organized into four parts, concerned with institutional closure, models of community services, the effects of deinstitutionalization on people with intellectual disabilities and, finally, the effects on families with intellectually disabled members.

INSTITUTIONAL CLOSURE AND REPLACEMENT

The first section of the book focuses on the closure of institutions and their replacement by services in the community. The first chapter in this group (Chapter 2) is by Donald Shumway, Director of Mental Health and Developmental Services for New Hampshire, the first American state to completely close its institutional care. Shumway gives a brief description of the closure of Laconia, the state's only institution, which illustrates both the range of processes involved and an evident commitment to improving services. Like many American examples, the closure of Laconia was undertaken by a coalition of parents, people involved in developing community services and also the people providing the institution. It used local and national law to drive the pace of change, and it involved a policy of leading through the development of community services until closure was obvious and inevitable, rather than of announcing closure as the starting point.

Paul Castellani, Director of Program Research for the State of New York Office of Mental Retardation and Developmental Disabilities, develops this picture in Chapter 3. He describes the progress of New York's plan to close all its institutions. Here the scale of the enterprise is much greater, involving 20 institutions serving 10 000 people. Castellani notes that extensive deinstitutionalization in the 1970s and 1980s has still not closed the institutions and that in order to achieve closure it was necessary to coordinate many different aspects of policy – especially in the middle of organizational hierarchies and at the boundaries between parts of the State government. Many factors other than ideological commitment had to come together to implement closure.

In Chapter 4 Jim Mansell, Director of the Tizard Centre at the University of Kent at Canterbury in England, describes work undertaken over a 15- year period to define and implement models of community-based supported housing services. The message here is that implementation of new services is problematic. Despite the successful demonstration of excellent client outcomes in services with explicitly planned approaches to organizing staff to meet individual needs, many ordinary community services seem to risk repeating institutional care practices. So, although great progress has been made in providing services in the community, these services often seem inadequate. Mansell notes that in the British context this appears to be linked to both the staff subculture in services and to questionable commitment to quality by decision-makers.

A similar problem is identified in Chapter 5 by Jan Tøssebro, of the Department of Sociology at Trondheim University, in the Norwegian context. The new local services set up in Norway since 1988 inherit many organizational features of the (small, well-resourced) institutions they replace. Although there is evidence of improvement in many aspects of service provision, Tøssebro cautions against expecting that deinstitutionalization will in itself undo or overcome the devaluation and stigmatization of people with intellectual disabilities and suggests that the new services themselves may one day carry the same connotations as institutions do now.

MODELS OF COMMUNITY SERVICES

In the next section of the book, three authors look at the models of community services that are developing in their countries. First, Kent Ericsson, Research Psychologist in the Department of Education at Uppsala University, describes the background to Swedish deinstitutionalization policy and the continuing struggle between institutional and personal frames of reference. After showing how the idea of normalization developed by innovators in the intellectual disability field had its roots in a wider political concern for social integration and solidarity and in the immediate post-war period, Ericsson develops the argument that a social and political commitment to people with intellectual disabilities as citizens with equal rights is a prerequisite for developing community services which really do give people a better life, and a stimulus to managers and staff of services to replace institutional responses with individually-tailored and negotiated solutions.

Mary Ann Allard, at the Centre for Social Policy Research at the University of Massachusetts at Boston, develops a similar theme in her description of the growth of supported living policies and programmes in the United States. Developing as a response to dissatisfaction with new community services which continue to have an institutional character, supported living offers a model of entirely individualized and flexible support which aims to avoid facility- or programme-based approaches. Allard notes that this idea is attractive not only because it offers the prospect of better services but also because it represents potentially more efficient use of resources at a time when social expenditure is under pressure; the situation in most western countries.

This section ends with a chapter by David Felce, Director of the Welsh Centre for Learning Disabilities in Cardiff, that looks inside the staffed house in the community and offers a model of the processes required to provide effective support for people with intellectual disabilities in the residential situation. Felce takes as his starting point the contrast noted by Mansell in Chapter 4 between demonstration projects and mainstream community housing in Britain. He describes the patterns of staff performance associated with good services and how they relate to features of service design and organization. He makes the point that simply changing features like size of group home (or even adopting new models like supported living) may not improve services if they fail to address the issue of how staff actually help the people they serve.

THE IMPACT ON SERVICE USERS

The third part of the book includes four chapters which bring together perspectives on the impact of deinstitutionalization in Finland, the United States, Britain and Norway, looking in particular at the outcomes experienced by people with intellectual disabilities themselves.

In Chapter 9 Timo Saloviita, of the Department of Special Education at the University of Jyväskylä, reports a study of relocation syndrome among people with intellectual disabilities moving out of institutions in Finland. This is a relatively neglected topic in intellectual disability and Saloviita makes links with the literature on studies of elderly people to inform the discussion.

James Conroy has been involved in a series of major evaluations of deinstitutionalization in the United States in recent years, beginning with the five-year study of the closure of Pennhurst carried out with Val Bradley (Conroy and Bradley, 1985). Now in private practice, he describes in Chapter 10 the results of an evaluation of the closure of institutions in Connecticut over the period 1985–90. This was a comprehensive study looking at many different indicators and the results add to the now substantial American literature showing overall benefits of moving from institutions to small-scale services in the community.

Eric Emerson and Chris Hatton, from the Hester Adrian Research Centre at the University of Manchester, have collected together the results of all the available studies of deinstitutionalization in Britain to produce a comprehensive overview, including material not previously published. In contrast to the American literature this shows a much more mixed picture in which, although community services generally produce better outcomes than institutional care, there is considerable variation within service type and the poorest community services appear no better on the measures studied than the institutions they were designed to replace. Emerson and Hatton also make the point, in contrast to Conroy's view of American experience, that there is little evidence of continuing improvement in British community services.

The last chapter in this group is by Johans Sandvin, of the Nordland Research Institute. He examines the implementation of the Norwegian reform and, echoing Tøssebro's findings in Chapter 5, finds a mixed picture of benefits and missed opportunities in the programme. Sandvin draws attention to an important aspect of recent Norwegian, Swedish and British reforms, which is the transfer of responsibility for services from central to local government agencies. He argues that one of the processes at work is 'dedifferentiation', through which people with intellectual disabilities experience both the benefits and the drawbacks of being given the same consideration as other people receiving local services.

THE IMPACT ON FAMILIES OF SERVICE USERS

The final section of the book also addresses the impact of deinstitutionalization, but now on the families of service users. In Chapter 13 Barbro Tuvesson, a social worker in Skövde in Western Sweden, and Kent Ericsson describe a study of the views of parents after closure of an institution in Sweden and the transfer of their relatives with intellectual disabilities to services in the community. The study shows that many parents were supportive of the change throughout, and that those people who had misgivings had these allayed, at least to some extent, once community services were operating. Where concerns were raised, however, they genuinely reflected problems in the organization of support in the community.

Jan Tøssebro (Chapter 14) uses a large survey in Norway to address the question of why parents oppose deinstitutionalization. The survey shows the same high levels of concern and scepticism before transfer apparent in the American literature. Tøssebro suggests that these views are primarily the product of two different factors. First, families are unclear about what is the alternative form of care in the community, not only because there are few new services to see at the outset but because the public authorities fail to clarify some of the organizational uncertainties involved. Thus, scepticism is not necessarily primarily about the ability or potential of people with intellectual disabilities but about the ability or potential of local authorities to do a good job. Second, Tøssebro suggests that families' main frame of reference is backward-looking and that the major improvements in Norwegian institutions in the 1970s are regarded as important, positive gains which further reform puts at risk.

In Chapter 15, Hilary Brown, Danuta Orlowska and Jim Mansell from the Tizard Centre at the University of Kent at Canterbury discuss parents' organizations in Britain. They point out that parents' organizations exist in a potentially problematic relationship to service users and to service organizations: that under some conditions (as in the Norwegian example) parents' concern to hold on to what they have already got may override their interest in supporting even better services. They suggest that a new research agenda needs to be constructed in partnership with parents, which attempts to understand the pattern of influence exerted on ordinary parents by services and their own élites to make them more or less compliant or difficult, conservative or radical.

Finally, in Chapter 16, Jim Mansell and Kent Ericsson attempt to draw some general conclusions about deinstitutionalization and outline some prospects for the future.

PART ONE:

Institutional Closure and Replacement

Closing Laconia 2

Donald Shumway

Since the end of January 1991, New Hampshire has provided services for people with developmental disabilities without any use of institutional care. It was the first state in the United States to have succeeded in closing all of its institutions for people with developmental disabilities. More recently, the District of Columbia and the State of Vermont have closed all institutional care. It has been my privilege to work on this project for 17 years, half of this time as its Director of Mental Health and Developmental Services. In this chapter a brief overview of the closure process at one institution is presented, highlighting some of the key processes and drawing out some guiding principles.

New Hampshire has adopted a commitment to helping restore citizens with all levels of disability, to being participating members of the communities of the state. The new services include very high levels of community-based work and individualized living arrangements. Although there is much to learn and a long way to go before this commitment to full inclusion and participation has been realized, the journey is off to a good start.

New Hampshire has 1.1 million residents. It is relatively small, being about 275 km north to south, and 175 km east to west. The more urban areas of the south have 900 000 people. In the north, New Hampshire is largely rural. Politically, it was well suited to replacing institutional care with services in the community. Symbolically, the licence plates for motor vehicles bear the slogan 'Live Free or Die'. Freedom is very important in the public consciousness of the people of New Hampshire. The politics of the state are considered generally conservative, often to the far right of centre. As a culture, New Hampshire was ready to debate the issues of confinement of people with disabilities, and consider freedom for each citizen, including the state's most disabled people.

CLOSURE OF LACONIA DEVELOPMENTAL SERVICES

Laconia was the only institution in New Hampshire, and its closure marked the end of 20 years' sustained effort. In 1970 the residential population of Laconia State School was 1200 people. Conditions were very bad. Facilities were 50 years old, staffing was minimal, and a pessimistic view of disability was the rule. The residents suffered greatly under these conditions (Figures 2.1 and 2.2).

In 1975 a collaborative effort of parents, who organized a chapter of the parents' Association for Retarded Citizens advocacy group at Laconia, and professionals working in state government, gained the passage of progressive legislation calling for:

- the establishment of an 'individual service plan' unique to each service recipient;
- services to be provided in the 'least restrictive settings' of the person's liberty;
- each service recipient to be granted the right to receive services of a quality which is the best that can be provided, to 'the limits of modern knowledge'.

The passage of legislation did not lead to prompt fulfilment of its promises. A few community services did begin though, and the number of people at Laconia began to decline. Conditions at the institution remained

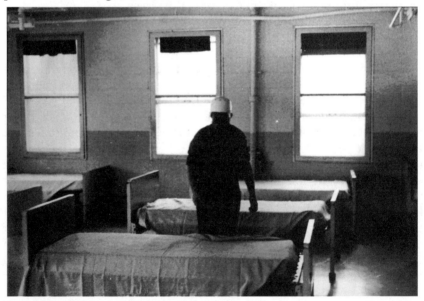

Figure 2.1 A ward in Laconia: interior.

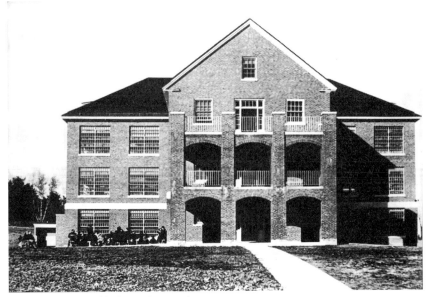

Figure 2.2 A ward in Laconia: exterior.

very poor for those who remained or were admitted. Parents and professionals continued to advocate for resources, eventually going to the
Federal Court in 1978 to seek an order for support of both the legal policies and funds necessary to carry out the legislation. In 1979, New
Hampshire experienced what, at the time, was the longest civil trial in its
history. Extensive public education was possible as a result of the trial.
The collaboration of professionals and parents continued with the positive result of the parents gaining a strong judicial order in 1981. The
Court's decree specifically and in detail required the state to carry out the
plans written by the State Division of Mental Health and Developmental
Services for developing a state-wide community support system. The
Laconia State School had to meet certain minimum standards and 235
individuals (a little less than one-half of the 620 people then in residence)
were projected to be placed in the community so as to allow Laconia to be
reduced to a size that, at the time, was thought to come close to the legal
standards. The Department of Education, also enjoined in the suit, was
required to provide local educational services to severely disabled children. While at the time questions were raised as to whether the court
should order the closure of Laconia State School, the court declined to
order that action.

In retrospect it seems likely that New Hampshire made the ultimate closure of Laconia easier by not outlining an actual closure plan. Even until the last six months of its existence, the State of New Hampshire did not state that its objective was to close Laconia State School. Instead, the objective was positive in its orientation to develop a comprehensive system of community services which would allow all individuals with developmental disabilities, regardless of the severity of their disability, to be provided for within community settings. Placements from the institution would occur person by person as required by state law and individual service plans. This focus on the positive development of a community service system and not on the negative proposal of closure, facilitated the ultimate closure by not polarizing the various parties: individuals, or families, or workers, or state departments, or the public on one side or the other of the philosophy of closure. The State of New Hampshire simply went about the business of developing opportunities for people with developmental disabilities, one by one, in their respective communities and made those services available to individuals at Laconia State School whose guardians and parents might choose to have them move to the community. Clients who were living at home were also given access to these new services. A person was placed from Laconia into the community only when all parties agreed that the supports were in place to make it a successful move. Only a very general schedule was needed; however, very intensive placement efforts were made.

It was only when approximately 30 people remained at Laconia State School and the institution yielded very poor economies of scale, that the high overhead for the single facility dictated that it ultimately be closed. Only then were the remaining individual families (who were the few families that had held back from considering community alternatives) urged in a final series of meetings between their Association for Retarded Citizens parent groups and the Division to allow placements and therefore the ultimate closure. During the last five years of its existence, no admissions were made to Laconia State School and in many respects, Laconia State School ceased to exist as an option for individuals and families in the community five years prior to its actual closing.

INSTITUTIONAL MANAGEMENT

The complicated process of closing the state facilities required an extraordinary degree of competent management throughout the service system, and that certainly included the superintendent and staff of the state facility. It required institutional leadership and staff dedicated to individuals moving into community services while providing high quality support for the clients who remained pending their placement. Staff at Laconia

State School were given repeated 'values' training such as PASSING, Social Role Valorization, and related instruction in normalization (Wolfensberger and Thomas, 1983; Wolfensberger and Glenn, 1975). Through this training they developed a strong commitment to the mission on behalf of individuals with developmental disabilities. A lot of time and money was spent on staff training but if we were doing this again, we would spend even more. The institutional staff were well meaning in their commitment to the clients, but they were not able to recognize and carry out dignified, individualized supportive care. Intensive values training developed a cadre of highly motivated staff who did know how to make the transition for themselves and their clients. This helped maintain staff focus and morale at Laconia which was essential to an orderly phase-out.

The best institutional staff had developed close personal relationships with many of the clients. As our experience grew, we creatively used those relationships in establishing individualized placements. As a result, as time went by some very interesting client service options have arisen. For example, several clients and staff have become co-tenants.

CONTROLLING COSTS

As we were converting institutional to community models through individualized placements, the phase-down of each institutional living unit was gradual. Many specific efforts were taken to assure each client of a non-frightening, supportive change process. Staff ratios of direct care and support staff (e.g. maintenance and food service staff) necessarily rose due to the needs of the remaining residents. To help control costs we periodically had to combine half-empty living units so as to close off buildings and reduce expenses. This was a difficult problem because clients sometimes were moved twice within the institution before their own placement. Likewise, staff had to learn the needs of new clients repeatedly in this process. This was a difficult trade-off between flexible schedules of community development through individual community placements, and the challenges of institutional operations. Our first priority had to be the careful development of community placements.

COMMUNITY SERVICES

As community-based residential services were developed in each local area, the opportunity was taken to incorporate case management and day programme services. Over 1200 clients now live in community residences and family support homes, and 200 clients live in supported independent living (Figure 2.3).

Our early community development efforts emphasized large group

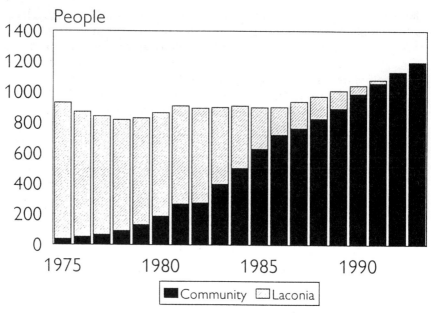

Figure 2.3 People living at Laconia and in the community 1975–93.

homes of eight beds, coupled with sheltered employment services or day activity programmes under the coordination of a case manager. By 1985 virtually all new developments instead became highly individualized with placements into settings where only one or two people with disabilities lived. Soon the eight-person group homes were being reduced to individual settings (Table 2.1).

A significant programme development was the emphasis on supported employment as the day programme of choice for adults with developmental disabilities. Many individuals leaving Laconia State School, as well as living in the community, were offered opportunities to participate in regular work places with non-handicapped peers and provided opportunities for integration in the work place that were both reinforcing and rewarding. The sheltered workshops also began to close.

New Hampshire also developed a comprehensive system of early intervention programmes for infants and toddlers, serving 1250 infants and families per year in 12 areas. Such early intervention programmes are the introduction to assistance and support for new families with children with developmental disabilities. These programmes were instrumental in serving families of children with developmental disabilities who might, in the past, have required institutional services.

More recently, we requested specific legislation to study the issue of

Table 2.1 Number of persons with a developmental disability in residential care by size of residence in New Hampshire

Size of residence	Number of persons		
	1986	1991	1993
1 person	27	291	334
2 persons	27	194	239
3 persons	36	162	227
4–6 persons	351	237	202
7–8 persons	261	129	83
9–12 persons	19	43	48
13+ (Laconia State School)	180	21	0
Total	901	1077	1193

family support. Families were brought together to design a family support programme. Families determined that each geographic area would have a programme governed by the families whose sons and daughters live at home with them. This has been a very successful action of empowering families to gain control over their lives. Three thousand, eight hundred families now receive flexible supports under the family support programme. Directed by local family support councils who plan and guide the family support staff, this process is also guided by a state level task force of families. We continue to search for ways to bring family/professional relationships back into balance throughout the service system.

These components – family support, integrated living, supported employment, early intervention, and public education – together ended the need for institutional placement at Laconia State School. The New Hampshire public began to develop a different perspective on the services that are most important for individuals with developmental disabilities. Most importantly, however, we have seen the institutional scars of severe self-abuse, bizarre behaviour, and dependence inflicted upon Laconia's residents giving way to engaged social connections and personal growth. We have also seen very high satisfaction levels by family members. Interviews with the 30 parents mentioned earlier as those 'holding out', who did not want community placements have since showed significant satisfaction levels with the new opportunities and experiences. Client satisfaction has also been very high.

RESOURCE ALLOCATION

These programme directions, and the significant cost of services led the State of New Hampshire, early in its developmental process, to choose two important financial policies.

Firstly, New Hampshire developed its service system based upon a model called individual financing for individual competency enhancement. Individual financing means that financial resources of the service system are assigned on an individual level, based upon that person's required support levels. The competency enhancement process permits us to continually pursue outcomes for individuals that allow them to use the competencies they possess so that they can work in integrated sites, live in integrated residential arrangements, and participate with their non-handicapped peers, using the skills that they possess and having those skills enhanced as a result of services provided under the funding that is assigned specifically to them. Tremendous capabilities for self-care and personal development have been revealed.

The second most important financial system that we have established concerned the transfer of institutional funds to follow the clients, with each building closure out into the community. This then set up an incentive as the community services tended to be less expensive than the final years of institutional care. Thus, we were able to serve many people who had never been institutionalized. In the later years, as the economy of the region suffered, the institutional budget also absorbed budget cuts. This was possible as we eliminated the very expensive and wasteful physical plant of the institutional campuses. Costs vary widely based on individual needs and the progress in personal growth that has occurred. After two or three years of community living, many clients have developed the skills and confidence to move to less structured living and work settings. With the shedding of the terrible behaviour patterns of institutional living, positive personal changes have led to stabilizing costs over the last several years. Nevertheless, we do still have a waiting list of 99 high priority clients.

THE FUTURE

Many families and professional colleagues in other states and countries have told us that the closing of Laconia Developmental Services is an important milestone of social change. This commitment to community participation by families and individuals with developmental disabilities has changed the face of New Hampshire communities and has changed opportunities for people with disabilities in extraordinarily significant ways. It is true that the size, affluence, culture, and homogeneity of the state presented certain unique opportunities for such change to more readily occur. Throughout this long process of transition for disabled people, three things stand out that are the most important; more essential than technical, managerial issues, and more fundamental than operational policy.

Firstly, the families have remained a strong, cohesive voice of constructive change. We owe a great deal to the support that all of the New Hampshire families have given. Throughout the most difficult days of budget threats, Federal court trials, policy debates, etc. the Association for Retarded Citizens and its families have stood as a strong voice for 'doing the right thing'. As a group of constituents, they have never become visibly fragmented into opposing camps. We have worked closely together and this has been crucial in managing the politics of change.

Secondly, my staff and that of our local agencies have shown great leadership and consistent commitment to the cause of aiding people with developmental disabilities in their quest for full citizenship, expertly managing the budget and policy of the community start-up and ably managing the phase-down of Laconia State School. They and many others have done all that was asked, days and nights, week after week, year after year. That consistency of dedication was and is indispensable in delivering on the promises, one by one, for our clients. In many ways we have been on a crusade, working closely as a group on behalf of a strongly held vision.

Finally, and most certainly, the true grit of the system has been in the quest for independence by the people with disabilities of New Hampshire. The risk taking has been first and foremost theirs. They have shown us that institutions were not created for their disabilities, but rather for our own inability to perceive and include their very real abilities. New Hampshire residents with disabilities are becoming contributing community members, taxpayers, and politically involved citizens. Recently one former Laconia resident was given the State's Martin Luther King, Jr Award for advancing the civil rights of all people in the state.

Is the job done? No, we have a long way still to go. In conclusion, I want to summarize certain valuable lessons we have learned.

- Values and beliefs come first: before technology, management structures, programme models and regulations.
- Lead the placement process with some of the most challenging clients: individuals whose behaviour presents a particular challenge and individuals with complex medical needs.
- Fight hard to keep people from having to return, once placed. This

involves setting up community options so that they have a very good chance of succeeding and sustaining staff's vision of ideal services.

- Work hard for family/client 'readiness' rather than skills readiness. The kind of readiness that matters is when families are psychologically poised for the change, based on their contact with successful services, values training, and security structures (give them the director's home telephone number).
- Highlight success stories: set a standard of excellence and use success to teach people how to make services work to achieve this standard.
- Bombard everyone with progressive ideas: use prominent national and local spokespersons and opinion leaders for families as well as for professionals, and build a local network or coalition of people who share the values of the new service.
- Quality measurement needs to promote success, rather than just focusing on shortcomings and it needs to include all aspects of service organization and provision.
- Carefully design individual transitions: do not focus on deficit/skills measurement, minimize the number of transfers, involve circles of support (friends and family) in decisions and dream dreams of new lives.
- Manage the process of change openly: give families/consumers/staff plenty of input and briefings on the status of the project and future plans and hold informal 'house meetings' – open invitation for consumers/families/staff at each institutional building and community region.
- Change occurs one person at a time: be individual centred, try things that have never been done before and be flexible.
- Look inside the local culture: allow the ordinary life experiences of your culture to become the model for the service system and take the best qualities of the culture and build on them.
- Assist people in personal growth: clients need to find ways to contribute to their world, and staff and neighbours need to establish newly balanced relationships, i.e. respect and friendship. Assist people in making real choices and having control over their lives.
- Institutions stereotype people with disabilities: find ways to see the individual, listen carefully, find ways for the individual to gain respected status and let control over resources and policy flow back to consumers and families.

New Hampshire now looks forward to a future of integration. Our mission remains:

> To create new opportunities for Granite State citizens with developmental disabilities. We shall work hard to promote the independence and integration of our neighbors with developmental

disabilities so that they can participate – right along side of non-handicapped people – in all facets of community life. We'll know we've been successful when there is evidence that people with disabilities are participating in their community, working at meaningful jobs, involved in integrated employment situations and enjoying the simple opportunities for life and recreation that the rest of the world takes for granted.

Closing institutions in New York State

3

Paul Castellani

In 1987, New York State announced that it would close six of its 20 large institutions for the care of people with developmental disabilities (largely mental retardation) by 1991. Coming on the heels of the 1984 decision to close Willowbrook Developmental Centre as the culmination of the long legal battle over that facility, this was a significant shift in the state's policy for the care of people with developmental disabilities. This would be the largest and most rapid closure of large institutions for the care of people with developmental disabilities in the United States. Toward the end of the first phase of closures in 1990, New York announced its intention to close all of its large institutions. By 1994, nine centres had closed, and there were less than 5000 people residing in the remaining facilities. New York was rapidly becoming the largest state to operate a system of services for people with developmental disabilities without large institutions. This was particularly important because New York's Office of Mental Retardation and Developmental Disabilities (OMRDD) had operated the largest system of institutions since the nineteenth century.

The decision to close these large institutions was a major new direction in the state's policy for the care of people with developmental disabilities, and their closure provided important lessons about policymaking and implementation in this area. This chapter examines both the decision to close and the implementation of the first phase of that policy.

THE DEVELOPMENT OF CLOSURE POLICY

DEINSTITUTIONALIZATION

Large institutions were historically major components at the core of service delivery for people with developmental disabilities in New York State (Rothman, 1971; Rothman and Rothman, 1984). Until approximately

15 years ago, services for people with developmental disabilities were provided either in these facilities or in small, largely parent-operated community programmes. Children with disabilities were routinely excluded from public schools, and there were no significant local government or private agency programmes. The large state institutions, called developmental centres in New York State, were the most visible and important providers of services.

In the late 1960s and early 1970s, against a backdrop of exposés of the appalling conditions in these institutions, a number of reforms began to take place (Castellani, 1987). Firstlyly, the principle of normalization emerged as a potent political ideology in the field. Adopted from Scandinavian theorists, it held that people with disabilities should live in circumstances as close as possible to the cultural norm for persons of the same age (Nirje, 1969; Bank–Mikkelson, 1969; Wolfensberger, 1972). Advocates for people with disabilities argued that large institutions were inconsistent with this principle.

Secondly, several pieces of landmark federal legislation in the 1970s began to lay the foundation for services and supports for people with disabilities in community situations. The 1975 Education of All Handicapped Children Act (PL94–142) mandated access to public schools. The Rehabilitation Act of 1973, with its Section 504, was also crucial in prohibiting the exclusion of people with disabilities from federally funded programmes.

Thirdly, a series of federal court decisions concerning the conditions of people living in large institutions had a major impact. In 1972 the Wyatt v. Stickney (344 F. Supp.387. M.D. Ala., 1972) case applied right to treatment standards to individuals living in large state institutions and mandated the State of Alabama (and others) to improve conditions. In the Willowbrook case in New York, ARC v. Rockefeller (72 Civ.356. E.D.N.Y., 1972), ultimately settled by consent decree, the state agreed to provide alternatives to institutionalization. In the Pennsylvania case of Halderman v. Pennhurst (446 F.Supp.1295, 1978), the federal district court expanded the remedies to include requiring the state to close the facility.

Finally, changes in federal regulations and funding had an important impact on the status of large institutions. Income maintenance through Supplemental Security Income and Social Security Disability Insurance provided substantial federal funds to underwrite the costs of community programmes (Braddock, 1987). Medicaid, a federal funding programme that reimbursed states for the cost of care of the aged and medically indigent, was passed in 1965. In addition to funding small Intermediate Care Facilities/Mental Retardation (ICFs/MR) in the community, in 1971 the federal government allowed states to designate large institutions as

ICFs/MR so that they could use the funds to improve conditions. This has had cross-cutting effects. The regulations that accompanied this large infusion of federal funds resulted in physical plant improvements as well as the hiring of larger professional and clinical staffs to meet the active treatment requirements that the medical model Medicaid entailed. It also required New York to move several thousand residents out of those facilities in order to meet the standards of space required for each person in the centre.

THE SPECIAL CASE OF NEW YORK

Closing institutions in New York is a particularly important example of policymaking and implementation because the centres had been rebuilt and revitalized during the 1960s and 1970s. During the 1960s, under the administration of Governor Nelson A. Rockefeller, New York embarked on an enormous public works programme. Several new developmental centres were built, and the existing ones were refurbished. Moreover, this programme was managed by new and expanded semi-independent public authorities that ultimately owned the buildings and bonded their construction. The mortgages on the buildings were largely financed by federal Medicaid reimbursement for the residents' services. Importantly, the salaries of a new cadre of young, professional, unionized state employees were substantially underwritten by the federal government through Medicaid. Although the institutions retained their physical appearance and distance from the community, several significant changes in their structure, financing, staffing, and role in a larger human services framework revitalized them in New York.

New York not only rebuilt, refinanced and restaffed its developmental centres with a large infusion of federal money, but it also used Medicaid to support its community programmes. In New York, ICF/MR funds were used to build small community-based facilities as well as finance the larger institutions. Additionally, New York converted a large number of its existing state-funded group homes to ICFs/MR, resulting in a 50% federal share of costs and increased professional staffing. It also used Medicaid funding to support many day services through its Day Treatment programmes. Of great importance in New York was the fact that in order to maintain Medicaid funding for the institutions, the state had to move several thousand people into community-based group homes in a relatively short period of time. This necessitated two crucial political and organizational strategies. Firstly, the state contracted with the advocacy and parent groups to provide many of those residential and day services, allowing them to fill approximately 50% of the places with people from their own waiting lists. Secondly, in order to maintain the political support of the state employee unions, the state established group homes and some day programmes using state employees. Consequently, deinstitutionalization proceeded with a critical political and organizational consensus between the private voluntary sector and state employees, both supported in increasing measure by federal Medicaid funding.

The collective impact of these factors in New York led to a programme of large-scale deinstitutionalization. Beginning in the late 1970s, New York, which operated the largest institutional system in the country, decreased the population in those facilities from over 25 000 in 1978 to fewer than 10 000 in 1987. Community programmes were developed for 17 000 former residents as well as people who had previously lived at home (Webb, 1988). Nonetheless, it is important to point out that deinstitutionalization was not closure, and until 1988, New York continued to operate 20 separate developmental centres (Castellani, 1992).

THE CONTINUING IMPORTANCE OF INSTITUTIONS

These factors were also important in those states that were undergoing deinstitutionalization. However, most states did not undertake deinstitutionalization on as large a scale as New York. Moreover, states remained very reluctant to close those facilities, and virtually all closures were the result of suits brought by advocates (Braddock *et al*. 1990). Where closures did occur they typically involved only one or two facilities at a time. In almost every instance these closures have been very problematic for the states in which they have been undertaken and have usually taken a number of years to accomplish (Bradley, 1985; Conroy and Bradley, 1985).

Nonetheless, the direction in the field was still moving towards developing community programmes, and the population in developmental centres declined. However, there were several reasons why these institutions continued to be important in the service system. Firstly, they typically housed the people with the most difficult problems, usually those with severe medical or behavioural problems. Many parents of residents of the centre were reluctant, cautious, or opposed to closure. Many of the specialized services in a local service system – particularly medical, dental and ancillary health services – remained in the large institutions. Most administrative and support services in the area also remained at the developmental centre. Even with the declining census in the New York facilities, the centre was still the largest concentration of employment in the local service system. While overall employment in a multi-county area might be maintained during deinstitutionalization, local government officials where the centres were located were very concerned about the dispersal of employment and its economic impact on the immediate community. Employees and their unions were concerned about the large-scale shifts in location and types of jobs that occurred in the transition from an institutional to a community programme service delivery system. Finally, the costs associated with operating the large institutions were important components in the overall federal reimbursement. While many argued that the costs of community programmes would be less than those of the institutions, state budget officials were very cautious about the implications for federal reimbursement of the transfer of costs from large facilities to community programmes.

THE RATIONALE FOR CLOSURE

As deinstitutionalization brought the institutions down to 10 000 in the same 20 centres, a number of factors moved the state towards closing them. There was a broad consensus that large institutions were not compatible with contemporary ideas about the housing of people with disabilities, and the extensive experience of deinstitutionalization demonstrated that people with the most challenging needs could live successful lives in the community. The role of the courts was another factor. Courts had already played an important role in New York State through the Willowbrook case, and the experience with judicial mandates was that they consumed inordinate amounts of time and attention as well as affecting virtually all staffing, resident movement, and programme decisions in the agency. A policy initiative favouring closure was therefore likely to forestall further court involvement.

The federal government brought increased pressure on New York State. Large institutions had become extraordinarily difficult environments in which to maintain the standards of care that were required by ICF/MR regulations. Not only was there an increasingly strong bias against large institutions, the growth in the ICF/MR programme became a focus of cost-cutting efforts by the federal government. The federal government's concern about its rapidly growing size and cost resulted in increased attention being given to the active treatment requirements of the regulations. The federal government began an aggressive programme of audits of New York's ICF/MR programmes seeking to disallow hundreds of millions of dollars of federal reimbursement paid to New York over the years. Akin to the problem with the courts, an increasingly large amount of New York State's attention had to be devoted to contesting the findings of the audits and meeting the standards to pass ongoing certification inspections. By far, developmental centres were the most troublesome element of this problem.

Deinstitutionalization also began to create problems of economy of scale for the developmental centres. A capital plan review showed that the costs of refurbishing large facilities for small numbers of residents would be ill-advised, especially since most of these residents would be moved out of the centre through the overall deinstitutionalization programme or as a result of court mandates. Additionally, the employment of a fixed number of institutional staff – such as grounds keepers, safety officers, power plant operators, and various building trade positions – became less and less cost efficient relative to that smaller number of residents. These factors began to appear more prominently in the analyses of budget and fiscal staff. These key actors were increasingly arguing that 120-bed developmental centres (particularly the older, larger ones) were inherently inefficient. In addition to the costs of institutional staff, deinstitutionalization also created imbalances in direct care and clinical staff-to-client ratios, and these were likely to result in layoffs of excess staff in the centres.

Deinstitutionalization had created an organizational and managerial capacity in the community which could be a foundation for closure. By 1987, over 500 voluntary agencies were providing services in New York State. In the three years prior to the closure decision, over 4100 new community residential places had been developed. In the five years prior to the closure decision, over 700 people each year had been moved out of the centres. By January 1987, the Office of Mental Retardation and Developmental Disabilities (OMRDD) and voluntary agencies were establishing community programmes at a rate of over 1500 residential beds and about 3000 day programme places per year (Castellani *et al.*, 1990). Creation of community programmes at this pace and scale involved setting up organizations, processes, and staff to undertake the increasing level of programme development. Additionally, a complex web of relationships was established with numerous other state governmental agencies, federal agencies, banks, and the myriad of other actors involved in this extensive undertaking. Over several years, formal and informal decision rules, routines, coordinating mechanisms, crisis management techniques, and a wide variety of other procedures emerged around the creation of community programmes. Additionally, the closure of Willowbrook, which the state had decided to close in 1985, was proceeding successfully. Issues of resident movement, community relations, alternative use of the campus, and transition of state employees to community jobs were all being dealt with to the satisfaction of key interests and political actors.

Deinstitutionalization resulted in a service system that, by 1987, was largely community-based although the large institutions continued to play important roles. A comprehensive network of private provider agencies had been established and state employees' jobs had been protected through the use of state-operated community programmes. Diseconomies in institutional capital plant and operations, the threat of lawsuits, problems of maintaining federal reimbursement for large facilities, and imbalances in staffing between institutional and community programmes had all pushed the state towards closure. The commissioner of OMRDD had a reputation as a 'policy entrepreneur' (Kingdon, 1987), and the state produced a broad-based policy to close six additional centres by 1991. To secure support for the policy, the state gave parents of residents strong assurances about health care in the community and reiterated its guarantee of employment to public employees. It also assured private agencies across the state that levels of community development would be maintained, and it got an enhanced, short-term reimbursement from the federal government to speed the closure of the centres. In many important respects, the closure policy was a large incremental step. Nonetheless, no other state had initiated as broad a policy on institution closure, one that would, and did, result in the decision to close all large institutions.

IMPLEMENTATION

New York State's experience is also important because it successfully implemented the closure decision, and this experience provided many important lessons in policy management and implementation. There is a large body of literature and experience that demonstrates that bold and innovative policy decisions are not self-executing (Levin, 1993), and New York State did indeed encounter a number of obstacles in its implementation.

THE 'NORMAL TURBULENCE' OF IMPLEMENTATION

Implementation of any significant policy initiative encounters 'normal turbulence' (Bardach, 1977; Castellani, 1992). Although New York had extensive experience of construction of community programmes, closure presented new challenges. Most of the problems were related to the simultaneous construction of so many new facilities in a short period of time. Timetables were shortened, and the usual problems that occurred tended to become crises. Those community groups that usually opposed construction of facilities in their neighbourhoods were able, in some locales, to take advantage of the situation to forestall construction. The other agencies involved in finance, approval of contracts, construction management, and other tasks found themselves often overwhelmed by the pace and scope of the construction programme. Moreover, closure of developmental centres did not proceed in an orderly, measured pace. There were often surges of demand for time, effort, and other resources – particularly towards the final stages – in each locale. In each instance, the key problem was to enlist other key actors and agencies for processing contracts, allocating funds, certifying new facilities, and completing the many other crucial tasks that were out of the hands of OMRDD. Construction stayed on schedule for the most part, but extraordinary efforts in crisis management and political pressure were often required.

A number of problems also occurred as OMRDD attempted to establish health and medical services in the community. In order to get the cooperation of parent groups, the administration had assured parents that the very high concentration of medical services in the centres would be maintained. Many of the problems of moving from a total institution to an integrated community approach to services occurred in this area. For example, in one district, a group home for medically frail, elderly people was constructed in a small town to take advantage of the hospital located there. One year after construction and relocation, the hospital was closed as a consequence of the state health department's policy to close small and inefficient hospitals. In another locale, OMRDD established its own mini-hospital by purchasing a defunct hospital in the community. In other closure districts, OMRDD instituted more typical arrangements for medical services by contracting with health maintenance organizations, medical groups, private practitioners, or by assisting the creation of private practices that would include people with disabilities by using purchase of service contracts with physicians who had previously been employed in the centres. Overall, integration into typical health settings of a large number of people who were perceived to be difficult to serve was an especially challenging aspect of closure implementation.

Another component of the closure policy was the commitment to ensure the jobs of the state workforce. An Employees' Services Office (ESO) was established to assist state employees in getting jobs in other state facilities or in the private sector. The ESO was originally established at Willowbrook where economic and organizational circumstances made assuring jobs a challenging task. The ESO model, with the original director, was transferred to the next closure site at Westchester. There, the refinement of the Employee Relocation Assistance Programme, a booming service economy in the area at that time, the close proximity of two other state institutions, and experience in the relocation task all encouraged a large number of employees – especially many in hard to recruit clinical positions – to leave the institution staff for similar or better jobs. The state then had to pay bonuses to try to temporarily retain these individuals so that minimum levels of staffing could be maintained. This problem resulted in some unanticipated costs, but the fiscal impact was minimal. Overall, however, the district directors had exceptional challenges in balancing, reconciling, and pacing the implementation of policies designed to close the institution as quickly as possible, maintain adequate staffing to meet standards of patient care, and ensuring that employees got jobs elsewhere. It was an indication of the problems that result from a poor fit between multiple policies and different environments.

IMPLEMENTING MULTIPLE POLICIES

These examples of normal turbulence and 'to be expected' problems demonstrated a crucial aspect of implementation. Like virtually all significant policy initiatives, the closure policy actually entailed several policies. Building community facilities, moving residents, protecting the jobs of state employees, developing health and medical services in the community, and converting institutions to alternate uses that would maintain adequate levels of state spending in the closure locales were among the major elements in the closure policy. Moreover, these had to be accomplished while sustaining previous levels of development in non-closure districts, maintaining the commitment to the private-sector agencies across the state, and carrying out other significant policy mandates such as the court-ordered placement of Willowbrook class clients. Ultimately, it highlighted the management difficulties involved in getting some degree of control over the implementation of distinct policies. It was not only a question of multiple policies but also the fact that key actors, often with indirect links to each other, had their own policy to implement and their own constituencies.

The inconsistencies within the overall policy and its lack of congruence with other policies created important implementation problems. On the one hand, they can be seen as a set of examples of the dynamic nature of implementation and the problems of coordination and control (Goggin *et al.*, 1990; O'Toole 1989). Problems arose as policymakers failed to know of or control which policies were being implemented or how those policies meshed with others, either within that particular initiative, with other agency initiatives, or with those of other government agencies.

There was also the important issue of how implementers not only managed a complex web of overlapping and often inconsistent policies but also made policy in significant ways. This occurred through a process in which implementation managers sorted out and selected which among the various 'policies' to implement and/or establish their own priorities among the multiple policy options. It also occurred when what appeared to be straightforward implementation management in one circumstance had important policy ramifications in another. New York's closure experience illustrated the need for implementers and policymakers to constantly revisit and adjust policy content, priority, and consistency as it changed in the implementation process.

MANAGING CHANGES IN POLICY

In addition to dealing with the multiplicity and inconsistencies inherent in major policy initiatives, implementation also had to contend with the fact that policies change. This was not a question of explicit revisions by the original policy actors but were the more subtle and complex changes that occurred over time, place, and circumstance that were particularly challenging to implementers because they were implicit, but nonetheless, significant (Bardach, 1977; O'Toole and Montjoy, 1984).

Firstly, new policy players entered the arena, and original players left. Implementation placed the key agency, OMRDD, in a web of relationships with several other state agencies, public authorities, local governments, private contractors, private voluntary agencies, banks, federal agencies, landlords and occasional other actors whose approval, cooperation, and/or involvement was necessary to complete the projects. Very early in the closure process, OMRDD was able to invoke the authority of the governor's office to resolve resource and timing problems in one district where the construction of a prison and high political visibility made meeting deadlines and commitments crucial. However, the ability to bring that authority to bear in relationships with other agencies tended to evaporate as closure implementation became more routine or involved less politically sensitive locales and circumstances. Moreover, the attention of executive office policymakers naturally shifted to other issues and problems over time, and the ability to intervene successfully in local political problems surrounding closure diminished. 'Recalcitrant agencies' (O'Toole and Montjoy, 1984) were able to become less visible to mandating authorities over time, especially since so many agencies were involved.

Not only did the priorities of the initial set of actors change, but the closure experience also demonstrated that the changing mix of policy actors who became involved as implementation unfolded had a substantial impact on implementation success. The possibility that a community facility being planned was on the site of ancient Native American burial mounds brought the state's historic preservation agency unexpectedly into the decision process. Problems with septic systems in group homes resulted in delays in getting certificates of occupancy from a local government as protracted negotiations with that county's health department took place. During the Mayoral primary campaign in New York City, properties seized by the city for unpaid taxes that had originally been promised as building sites were not turned over to the state because one candidate – who also held a key position in the city administration – was apparently concerned about the political ramifications of the decision. These are just a few examples of how new actors entering into the implementation process brought changes in the mix of players and priorities as well as new policy issues that had to be resolved.

Changes in the fiscal climate and problems encountered as implementation moved from one locale to another were other instances of these subtle, but nonetheless difficult, changes in policy. Over the period of implementation, the state's fiscal situation worsened dramatically. The state's ability and willingness to devote additional resources to resolve an implementation problem, for example, by paying contractors bonuses for early completion, diminished. Many of these latter effects of fiscal austerity were fairly easy to see. Less evident, but also very problematic, was the general caution that became pervasive as actual or anticipated freezes and cutbacks affected virtually all of the agencies and actors in the large interorganizational landscape of closure implementation. Contract processing slowed, commitments of staff time lessened, and willingness to take risks diminished. All of these apparent and subtle changes in the fiscal climate had important negative impact on closure implementation even though the policy was designed to carry the overall commitment through these cycles of fiscal well-being.

Policy implementation also varied significantly across locales. What worked in upstate New York did not work as well in New York City. There were fewer community resources, especially health-related services in New York City on which to build programmes. The financial instability of some community voluntary agencies slowed development. The shift from one locale to another not only involved dealing with different resources and needs but also a shift in the political context of implementation. For example, the relationships among parents, employees, provider agencies, neighbours, local government officials and community leaders, state representatives, and the state agency district directors were significantly different between the upstate, more rural locales that were the focus in the early stages of closure and those in New York City that came later. In upstate locales most of the programmes that were set up to achieve closure were state-operated and located in small communities where local governments, businesses, and community leaders usually welcomed the economic impact of even a small number of group homes and day programmes. Moreover, the district director, as one of the largest employers in the area, usually played an important and visible role in community affairs. In New York City, private agencies played the major role in operating residences and day programmes and had important independent ties to political and community leaders. Aside from a few instances where a planned development created a problem (e.g. on the site of a vacant lot that was a neighbourhood garden), the neighbourhoods in New York City seemed less aware and concerned about economic impact. However, where community awareness, opposition, or demands for more services did arise, planning district, borough, city, and school district politics were more complex and often more intense than that found in most upstate communities. As problems arose and engaged local government actors and agencies, the state agency and its district managers had much less political leverage in New York City than they enjoyed in upstate communities.

POLICY AND IMPLEMENTATION LESSONS

The success of the 1987 decision to close seven developmental centres can be gauged in two ways. Firstly, all of the centres did indeed close. One of the largest closed two years earlier than the original plan, and the last two centres in New York City closed a few months after the original deadlines. All of the major policy objectives on establishment of community services, movement of residents, transition of staff to jobs in the community, and alternative use of the institution were met. The secondly measure of the success of the 1987 policy was the decision to close all large institutions in New York State by the year 2000. This decision came in 1990 towards the end of the firstly phase of closures and was broadly supported by parent and advocacy groups, public employee unions, and all other major interest groups and political actors. This experience has several important policy and implementation lessons.

POLICY LESSONS FROM THE NEW YORK EXPERIENCE

New York's decision to close six large institutions in addition to the already announced closure of Willowbrook was a significant new direction in public policy in this area. Closure had circulated in the 'primeval soup of policy' (Kingdon, 1987) for some time. Several states had already closed some facilities, and other closures were underway. However, no state had embarked on a closure policy as broad and far-reaching as New York's. In contrast to the situation in virtually all states with lengthy, court-ordered closures, New York's administration was unique in initiating a broad policy to close one-third of its institutional capacity in five years. Moreover, it was apparent to most key actors that the successful closure of these facilities would quickly lead to the closure of all large facilities. While there were many philosophical, operational, and fiscal problems associated with running large institutions, closure was not a foregone conclusion. The fact that almost all states, with the exception of three of the smallest (New Hampshire, Rhode Island and Vermont), continued to operate large institutions indicates the magnitude and distinctiveness of New York's decision.

New York's decision had a very sound foundation. Ten years of large-scale and rapid deinstitutionalization had put several key elements in place. State-operated as well as private agency-operated community services provided the vehicle to deal with the critical issue of institution employees. The community system of residential and day programmes provided an already existing base of programmes. Large-scale deinstitutionalization had established managerial capacity and experience throughout important implementing agencies, administrative units, and district offices that would also be critical to closure. The experience of staff, parents, and residents with community programmes had also created a broad base of positive expectations that would carry over to closure. The Willowbrook experience on workforce, alternate use, and community relations showed the Governor's Office and other key policymakers that OMRDD could successfully deal with politically delicate issues.

But deinstitutionalization was not closure. New York's unique experience demonstrated the necessity of pulling these forces and factors together into a coherent closure policy and strategy. The possibility of litigation and federal action continued to pose threats to the autonomy of OMRDD and the state to manage its system of services. Less apparent but more immediately problematic were the increasing imbalances and anomalies that deinstitutionalization had created in OMRDD's budget structure. With the fiscal experience of OMRDD's executives and the propensity for innovation on the part of the commissioner, OMRDD was able to craft a policy that got the endorsement of the governor. It was also able to put into place other critical elements on workforce, alternate use, and community resources that allowed it to quickly sell that policy to key constituents.

The major elements of the closure policy also placed it in the state's overall developmental disabilities policy context. The policy conveyed several crucial messages. Closure would be a new initiative that would not displace a variety of existing commitments. In addition to judicially mandated obligations, commitments to the private voluntary agencies, to those interested in development in non-closure districts, to parents and consumers, to state employees, and to local governments and businesses were made and reiterated. The very good fiscal position of the state in 1987 provided an impetus and plausible setting for these commitments.

The decision to close several large institutions was a very important new direction for public policy for New York, and it showed a new course for policy in this area for other states. Its rationale, shape, scope, and direction provided significant lessons for policymaking. Moreover, the forces that led to the closure decision, the residual factors that undergirded institutions, the elements of the policy, the roles of key actors and interests, the processes and mechanisms used to put the policy together, and its timing all continued to be important factors in the implementation of the decision.

IMPLEMENTATION LESSONS FROM THE NEW YORK EXPERIENCE

New York was successful because in addition to the underlying political consensus in favour of closure, it had also established the organizational capacity and managerial experience to implement the decision. Nevertheless, closing seven large facilities more or less simultaneously was a very large and complicated management task. It involved several distinct dimensions, and substantial failure in any one of the areas would have critically impaired closure. OMRDD was particularly well situated to implement closure of several facilities. It had managed a very large and rapid deinstitutionalization that involved many of the same issues, mechanisms, and capacity in the public and private sectors that would be encompassed in closure. However, closure brought about its own problems and opportunities in several key areas.

From the perspective of success in implementing closure, there was probably little adjustment in policy design that would have significantly lessened the problems encountered. The schedules might have been lengthened, and closures could have taken place more sequentially than simultaneously. Nonetheless, the problems of implementing change, multiple and complex policies, the erosion of support on the part of top policymakers, the changes in the mix of policy actors, and the changes in context that had substantial impact on closure implementation would have remained. Overall, experience in implementation does indeed provide lessons for policy design. But in each specific case, the interplay between policy and implementation is complex (Nakamura, 1987). The ways in which the actions of implementers made policy and the failure of policymakers to adequately take this into account as implementation unfolded obviously created problems for policy and management. As Lynn (1981) pointed out:

Policy significance impregnates decisions and actions taken at all levels; high, middle, and low. Political executives who would be concerned with policy making must be concerned with activities taking place above, besides and below them, with games at all levels. Policy making is virtually indistinguishable from public management.

(Lynn, 1981, p.157)

The closing of institutions showed that policymaking occurred throughout the implementation process. Not only did implementers make policy, but policy preferences shifted over time and circumstance, and new policy actors with different preferences became involved in significant decisions affecting closure. There was a substantial and reciprocating linkage between policy and management throughout implementation. Looking more closely at the problems that arose from this permeation of policy and management, the role of managers emerged as crucial. Policymakers change more frequently, their interests naturally shift to other problems, and their ability to sustain involvement in implementation can be expected to erode. Managers, on the other hand, tend to have more long-lasting and stable involvement in the issue. Moreover, as the closure experience demonstrated, managers played subtle but important roles in making policy as implementation unfolded. The role of policy design and that of policymakers in implementation is crucial. But, to more fully appreciate the importance of cases like New York's where policy design was not fatally flawed and the role of policymakers in implementation was largely what one should expect, it is more important to focus on the role of management in implementation success.

Firstly, more attention must be paid to management capacity, especially policy management capacity. Secondly, it is important to recognize the crucial role of middle managers in implementation success. Thirdly, more attention must be paid to the importance of the interorganizational aspects of policy management. Taken together, they also point to new perspectives that should enhance our appreciation of the elements of implementation success.

The elements of management capacity

Change was the factor that presented the most problems in implementation; changes in policy and changes in context. Firstly, the problems encountered in managing the complex and fluid relationships in closure forces us to reconsider the management capacity on which the policy, in large part, rested. Studies of local government management capacity point out that management capacity actually consists of three distinct types of capability: policy management, resource management, and programme management (Burgess, 1975; Gargan, 1981). Gargan (1981) points out that each of the three management areas involves different participants. Moreover, Gargan (1981) also observes that 'the actual level of capacity is also determined by the context', and 'capacity levels may shift over time as a result of changes in the context rather than changes in specific management techniques'.

Managing the middle game

A secondly important issue is where to focus concern for policy management. The notions of 'policy' are usually associated with state-wide executive and legislative actors. The game metaphor has long been used in the study of implementation (Bardach, 1977), and a slight modification of Lynn's (1981) use of the 'high, low, and middle games' metaphor provides a perspective on where the problems of implementing closure occurred and where we must look for their resolution to the problems of policy management in the future. That is, if we view policy management as the capacity to bridge the strategic and routine, then a large portion of the burden for implementation success falls on middle managers. The definition of 'middle management' is elusive and always subject to shifts depending on the cast of characters. In closure implementation, the district directors and their top staff played crucial middle management roles between the overall policy decisions made at the state-wide level on closure and the tasks of dealing with local governments, parent and community groups, unions, provider agencies, contractors and other actors in acquiring properties, overseeing construction, negotiating contracts and the myriad of other tasks involved in closing the developmental centres and opening community programmes. In this context, the policy management capacity of middle managers was crucial to implementation success. So, what do middle managers need to know and do in order to achieve success in this fluid and complex environment of policy and management?

Policy management at the seams of government

Here, we have lessons learned in the past but perhaps forgotten. Virtually all of the major problems that did occur in implementation took place at 'the seams of government' reinforcing the importance of recognizing the intergovernmental and interorganizational aspects of implementation (Elmore, 1986). Thompson speaks of a 'mosaic of implementation' combining strategic considerations and bureaucratic routine (Thompson, 1984, p.148). Weiss (1987) argues that interorganizational relationships are a series of events and stages that unfold over time rather than a static set of go/no-go calculations (Weiss, 1987, p.113). These surges of demand, unpredictable patterns of interaction over time and place, as well as a natural waning of attention as implementation progressed were especially confounding. Many of these factors were contextual and may have overwhelmed management capacity in some instances. Nonetheless, Agranoff's (1986) notion of 'intergovernmental management' points to the ongoing problem-solving orientation required of those who work at the margins between organizations which characterized so much of closure implementation. These webs of relationships encompassed virtually all permutations of organizations on any particular issue rather than the more predictable pattern of intergovernmental and public–private sector relationships that characterize much of the literature on implementation. Being able to successfully deal in a world of temporary coalitions, task groups, and other 'adhocracies' rather than the formal mechanisms of intergovernmental and public–private relations are crucial to success in this area. Agranoff (1986) also emphasizes the importance of an appreciation of the political nature, in both partisan and interorganizational aspects, of the tasks of intergovernmental management. Problem-solving, negotiation, and conflict resolution are skills more important in this arena than the routine management capacity and technical competence we usually associate with middle management. These perspectives provide a managerial complement to the observations about the nature of linkages among organizations and their relationship to the context of implementation. That is, they indicate that flexibility, authority, and a set of skills not usually associated with the supervisory and routine roles of middle management are crucial. The capacity to manage changing relationships in a fluid environment are qualities required of managers in successful implementation. These aspects of management capacity have not been adequately integrated into our understanding of implementation success.

Overall, the closure experience points to two conclusions about managing implementation. Firstly, a fuller understanding of the interplay between policy and implementation should enhance our appreciation of the large burden placed on managers and the importance of the policy management component of management capacity. Secondly, this burden falls heavily on middle managers as they operate at the seams of government. This suggests that the orientation, skills, and techniques of intergovernmental management become much more important for implementation success.

CONCLUSION

The success of the 1987 policy which led to the decision to close all of New

York's developmental centres was based on its implementation. While deinstitutionalization established crucial elements of organizational and managerial capacity, deinstitutionalization was not closure. Closure involved the management of a number of distinct dimensions which were often inconsistent or incompatible. Moreover, all the other policies at work within the developmental disabilities arena had their own force and direction. In the best of times, which prevailed in 1987, there were significant difficulties in reconciling and coordinating them with closure. As the fiscal climate changed for the worse, and the attention of top policymakers moved on to other issues, and other elements of the context of closure became more difficult implementation became an even greater challenge. The ability of policy managers working at the seams of government was a critical factor in this success.

There are a number of lessons from the closure of large institutions in New York State. Overarching the particular lessons, however, was the demonstration of the residual strength of institutions. No matter how small they became during deinstitutionalization and then closure, they exerted enormous conceptual and organizational force throughout the process. The perceptions of parents, residents, employees, administrators, and the general public continued to be shaped by reference to the institution as the hub of services in a locale. In many respects, closing became more difficult towards the end of the schedule as the most persistent problems remained, and the experience of institutional solutions lingered. Of special significance was that New York's large institutions were not atrophying remnants of an earlier era. New buildings, new sources of funding, links to other institutional systems, and young, professional, and well-paid employees made them powerful organizational, political, and economic entities at the state and local levels. New York's success in creating a policy to close those institutions was based on a recognition of the needs of the various constituencies in the political and economic consensus that undergirded them. New York's ability to produce a closure policy was also largely due to the fact that deinstitutionalization had brought the service system to a point where a policy initiative was an important incremental reconfiguration of services. A few years ago, New York State operated the largest system of institutions in the world. One-half have closed, less than 50% of the peak census remains, and all large institutions in New York State will be closed in a few years. Closing large institutions put New York State in a position to move towards providing more typical forms of access to services and supports for people with developmental disabilities.

Issues in community services in Britain

4

Jim Mansell

In this chapter, I want to consider the way in which British community services are developing as institutions are closed. Firstly, I will survey the development of community-based residential services in our own work and the results of their evaluation. Then I will comment on the factors we think might be important in explaining their performance and illustrate one attempt to tackle them. Finally I will draw attention to some limitations of this and other work and suggest some possible future implications for service development in Britain.

Since the early 1980s my colleagues and I have been working with health and social service agencies in south-east England on the development of staffed housing as a replacement for institutional care of people with severe and profound learning disabilities.

In Britain, staffed housing (or supported housing, or staffed group homes) typically consists of a house (more rarely an apartment) for a small group (2–6 people, up to 7 or 8 in older services) of service users, supported by a team of staff. These schemes have mainly developed for former residents of institutions. Some of them are organized as residential services in which the house is owned by the service agency (a health authority with or without institutions to run as well, or a local authority social services department), which employs the staff (who may include professional qualified nurses or social workers but who increasingly are likely to have no formal qualification). In other cases the housing may be provided by another organization, giving the service user the status of tenant or licensee and separating the staff support and accommodation functions; the staff may be employed by a not-for-profit agency, and may be called 'house companions' or 'support workers' rather than 'care assistants'; they may be organized as a team supporting a number of people in different placements rather than being attached to one building.

These services are often funded through imaginative combinations of individual social security benefits and agency service expenditure (which are generally not permitted to be combined). The costs of these services are usually more than the average costs of institutional care: this is in contrast to the United States, Sweden and Norway where it appears that institutional improvement brought costs up to levels comparable with or exceeding community services (Chapters 1, 3 and 5).

Apart from a reducing amount of public institutional care (Chapter 1), the main alternative to this kind of residential service in Britain is care in private-sector residential homes which are typically larger, with lower staffing levels, funded from social security contributions and which may replicate many features of institutional organization. Present British government policy explicitly permits a wide range of types of residential care (National Health Service Management Executive, 1992; Department of Health, 1992) and although in some parts of Britain (e.g. Hampshire) 25-place units have been closed in favour of staffed housing, in others (e.g. Clwyd) institutions closed by the public sector are reopened as private homes.

THE MODEL OF CARE IN STAFFED HOUSING

The staffed housing model we have used was based on earlier work in Wessex (Mansell *et al.*, 1987; Felce, 1989). The key feature of this model is that, in addition to providing a well-staffed setting in ordinary housing in the local community of the people served, particular attention is paid to the way staff organize their work with service users. The aim is to help the people served take part in all the activities of daily living, instead of the typical arrangement where staff do all the housework and create large amounts of free time which they then find difficult to fill with constructive therapeutic activity (Chapter 8). To adopt this approach with people who have profound learning disability and who may have other problems such as challenging behaviour requires that staff break down activities into parts that people can do, and then provide only just as much help as is needed to keep the flow of client engagement going (Brown and Bailey, 1987; McGill and Toogood, 1993). Activity organized in this way then provides a realistic context for incidental teaching and for the ongoing management of problem behaviour.

A service organized on this model ought to be able to achieve higher levels of participation in meaningful activity than otherwise, broadening the experience of service users and increasing the possibility of growth and independence. And this indeed was the case. A series of studies by Felce and his colleagues (Chapter 8) showed markedly higher levels of engagement in meaningful activity (Felce *et al.*, 1985; Felce, de Kock and Repp, 1986; Thomas *et al.*, 1986), increase in adaptive behaviour (Felce, de Kock, Thomas and Saxby, 1986) and more social integration (de Kock *et al.*, 1988; Saxby *et al.*, 1986) when compared with people in institutions or large hostels.

Although government policy in Britain did not explicitly embrace the staffed housing model of residential care, the deinstitutionalization movement created favourable conditions for staffed housing to grow. The government 'Care in the Community' initiative (Knapp et al., 1992) promoted community services (albeit not necessarily for the most disabled people nor in small homes); the independent King's Fund Centre vigorously promoted the idea of 'An Ordinary Life' (King's Fund Centre, 1980); and the Campaign for People with Mental Handicaps introduced Wolfensberger's ideas about normalization through the medium of workshops on 'Program Analysis of Service Systems' and its derivatives (Wolfensberger and Glenn, 1975; Wolfensberger and Thomas, 1983).

In south-east England we were able to achieve widespread dissemination of the staffed housing model in the mid-1980s through a training initiative for people involved in closing Darenth Park and other institutions (Mansell, 1988a; Mansell, 1988b; Mansell, 1989). Figure 4.1 shows the number of staffed houses set up by health authorities (i.e. excluding social services and independent agencies) in the four London regions (covering a total population of about 13 million) from 1980–86; it shows that all the regions had begun to develop staffed housing by 1986 but that in the south-east there was a much greater increase.

Our optimism about the potential of this model of care meant that, when the regional health authority asked for help in deciding how to serve people in the institutions who were regarded as impossible to manage in the community because of their problem behaviour, we were able to persuade them to set up specialized staffed houses, at least for people with severe and profound learning disabilities. Recognizing the lack of expertise in developing sufficiently well-organized and structured community services, the authority funded us to set up a 'Special Development Team' to help local agencies. Using a process of individual service planning coupled with extensive practical help and some transitional financial incentives, the Team helped establish and support community placements (McGill *et al.*, 1994, Emerson and McGill, 1993; Toogood *et al.*, 1988). The Team focused on people with severe or profound learning disability (a separate initiative was proved for people with mild or moderate learning disability). Each specialized staffed house was individually planned for one or two people regarded as being the most difficult to serve in the community, living with people with less severe disabilities in a staffed

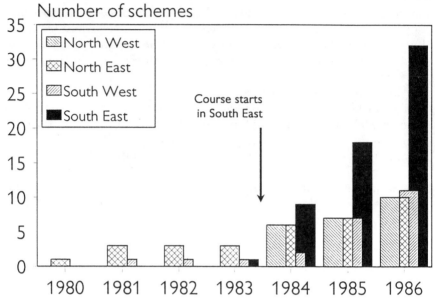

Figure 4.1   Number of staffed houses provided by health authorities in metropolitan regions 1980–86.

house or apartment. In most cases the plan was for one person with serious problem behaviour to live with 1–3 other people with mental retardation but without such serious problem behaviours or complex medical needs which might require the immediate attention of staff.

Evaluation of these services also showed marked improvement over the institutional services in which people formerly lived. On transfer, individuals increased their level of participation or engagement in meaningful activity by between one-third and over six times their average baseline level (Figure 4.2). As well as more leisure and self-care activities, individuals joined in household and community activities such as gardening, shopping and housework. Where pre- and post-transfer data on adaptive behaviour was available it showed marked increases (of 24–98%) in all but one case (Figure 4.3). Although the people concerned were selected as having the most serious challenging behaviour, these good results were achieved without any overall increase in challenging behaviour. The pattern of interaction from staff was much more supportive than in the institutions, with significantly higher levels of social contact and practical assistance: in terms of added value, the houses had just over double the staff:client ratio of the hospitals and special units, but they delivered 3.4 times the staff contact and 4.5 times the assistance to the individuals served. They were therefore able to use the greater resources

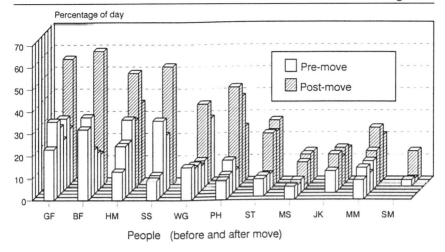

Figure 4.2 Percentage of day spent engaged in constructive activity before and after transfer to small staffed houses.

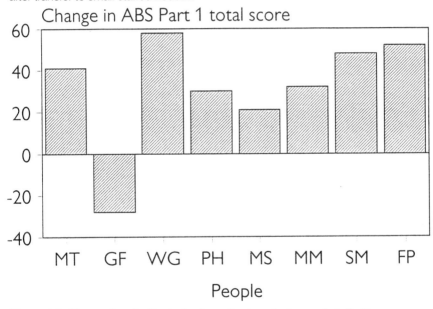

Figure 4.3 Change in adaptive behaviour after transfer to small staffed houses.

they had more efficiently, and this had greater effectiveness in terms of client participation in meaningful activity without overall increases in problem behaviour (Mansell and Beasley, 1993; Mansell and Beasley, 1990; Mansell, 1994; Mansell, 1995).

These quantitative data are supported and extended by qualitative accounts of the improvements in quality of life experienced by some of the service users involved (Felce and Toogood, 1988; Di Terlizzi, 1994).

Thus, both in the earlier work in Andover and in the Special Development Team project in south-east England, it has been possible to demonstrate the achievement of very good outcomes for service users, including people with severe or profound learning disabilities and additional problems of serious challenging behaviour, in staffed housing.

'MAINSTREAM' STAFFED HOUSING

At the same time, there have been several studies of 'mainstream' staffed housing services in south-east England which present a rather more mixed picture. Figure 4.4 summarizes the results of a number of studies of client engagement in meaningful activity (these form a subset of those used in Chapter 11). The methods used in these studies differ in detail, but are sufficiently similar to enable worthwhile comparisons to be made. While two studies carried out by psychologists working in services show comparable average engagement to the Andover and Special Development Team evaluations, our own studies found much lower engagement, comparable to that found in some local institutions.

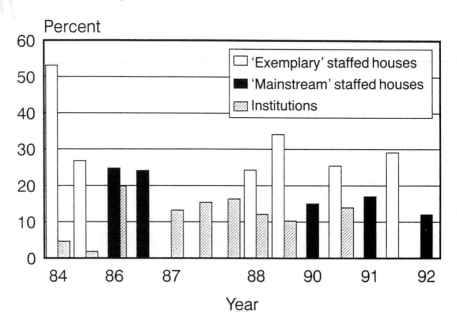

Figure 4.4 User engagement in constructive activity in recent studies.

A rather similar picture emerges if one looks at the percentage of time staff contact the people observed. This despite much higher staffing levels in houses than in institutions. Similarly mixed results may be beginning to emerge in relation to adaptive behaviour. Whereas two studies have reported gains in adaptive behaviour in staffed housing (Lowe and de Paiva, 1990; Felce, de Kock, Thomas and Saxby, 1986) another has not (Beswick, 1992).

Even though there may be other benefits of living in the community (such as better family and community contact), engagement in meaning-ful activity and adaptive behaviour are such central measures of quality that poor results deserve attention. It is clear that they are not due to gross differences in the characteristics of the people served, nor in the staffing ratios provided.

These mixed results are in contrast to the impression gained from pub-lished American research of consistent evidence of improvement in community services (Chapter 10). Although most of that research focuses on adaptive behaviour rather than engagement in meaningful activity the two ought to be related: if people are increasing their skills to the extent that it can be measured on a rating scale, surely this must mean they are participating to a greater extent in meaningful activity (i.e. behaving more independently). This discrepancy would be worthy of further study.

In the British context, where there is no clear policy commitment in favour of non-institutional services, these kind of mixed results are poten-tially very damaging in weakening the case for investment in new models of care.

THE REASON FOR MIXED RESULTS

UNCLEAR GOALS AND LACK OF DIRECTION

We have been able to explore the reasons for these mixed results in three studies of staffed housing services where agencies provide 10–20 staffed houses. These agencies are not necessarily representative in that they are all in London and our involvement has been prompted because they faced particular problems. One was a health authority with whom we worked on problems of placement breakdown (Mansell, Hughes and McGill, 1993); another was a not-for-profit agency set up collaboratively by health and social services and the third was a social services department.

All three showed evidence of unclear goals and lack of direction. Although goals are often related to normalization principles we have found that staff get little guidance on the interpretation of these princi-ples in practice. Values may be clearly communicated to them but how these should be operationalized is not. Thus, for example, we have found the situation where people with profound learning disabilities are denied participation in everyday activities because these are not seen as sufficiently intrinsically interesting or status-bearing by staff, who nevertheless cannot arrange enough of such opportunities to avoid individuals spending long periods doing nothing. Similarly, we reported an instance (Mansell and Beasley, 1990; 1993) where staff made complex verbal requests of non-verbal clients because they believed that this was properly respectful, and took non-response or initial withdrawal to mean that the person was choosing not to take part. They rejected advice to temper their acceptance of such choices with efforts to broaden client experience and shape up a history of successful participation.

Failure to specify clear goals for staff work with clients contrasts with the power with which organizations demand results in relation to bureaucratic procedures. So another common finding is that the home leader, who should be the principal teacher and guide of the care staff, becomes an administrator. This was an early finding of the research into the first generation of community units in Wessex (Felce *et al.*, 1980) and remains depressingly common. In one of the services studied a home for eight people had 72 different types of form or record in use, of which only seven related directly to service users. This imbalance in the weight attached to bureaucratic issues rather than meeting the needs of the people served may also lead staff to doubt the importance of the latter or to be unduly influenced by what guidance is present and clear rather than what the situation demands. In this house, for example, there is no written guidance for staff about how to organize activities so that people can join in even if they are prone to problem behaviour; but there are six pages of precise instructions on how much force, restraint and detention could legally be used with a resident.

INSUFFICIENT PREPARATION AND HELP FOR STAFF

There is evidence that staff in community services experience greater role ambiguity than insitution staff (Allen *et al.*, 1990). Their job has more components, their job title is less clear and the tasks are more sophisticated. In these circumstances, training is particularly important. However, a lower proportion of staff in community services are likely to be formally trained than in institutions in Britain. This is partly because attempts to reform and integrate nursing and social care training at the beginning of the 1980s were thwarted by the nursing unions and partly because current government policy denies that residential care in the community is a professionally skilled job (Griffiths, 1988).

In none of the three services we have studied has there been effective induction and in-service training reaching everyone who needs it. Figure 4.5 summarizes the training received by a sample of 26 staff interviewed (1 in 4 of the total staff) in one of these services. This service claimed an active training programme yet one-quarter had not had any induction training in the first six months of work and about three-quarters had not had any training in skill-teaching or managing problem behaviour. In another, service staff identified as a key issue that their training was heavily values-based and did not include sufficient practical work to enable them to translate these values into practice.

Thus, these community services are being set up without a cadre of well-trained staff at team leader level and with many striking gaps in the training offered to the unqualified staff in the team.

Training is only likely to be effective where it is supported by management leadership. A recent study in another part of south-east England has shown that staff feel that management's true objectives are not congruent with the espoused care objectives and that trained behaviour deteriorates quickly at work (Freeman, 1993). Even if this were not so, evidence from our own work suggests that there is an inverse relationship between seniority and competence at hands-on work with clients, so that just as house leaders become less skilled and less involved in work with clients because they spend less time with them so their managers are even less use as role models.

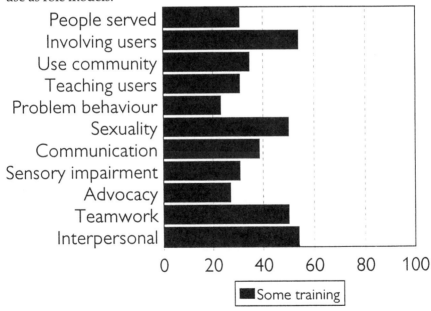

Figure 4.5 Percentage of staff trained in key areas.

British services are also increasingly generic in their organization, so that the first or second tier above the residential staff group is likely to be someone with responsibility for other client groups too, who may not have any expertise in serving people with learning disabilities. This is part of the problem of 'dedifferentiation' described by Sandvin (Chapter 12). When services for old people are heavily dependent on large, institutional residential homes, and when mental health services remain dominated by medical models, it is much more difficult to sustain a radical vision for learning disability services among managers responsible for all three.

ABSENCE OF MONITORING AND ACCOUNTABILITY

Since we have found that these services do not clearly articulate some important practical goals for the quality of care they provide, nor do they train staff in the working methods needed, nor do they use managers to model good practice in work with clients, it is perhaps not surprising that they do not monitor these things nor hold people accountable for them. In fact, they tend not to notice them until a crisis occurs. Even when crises do occur, they are now represented as evidence of individual failures by staff or managers or organizations, rather than as evidence of systemic processes; it is as if the hard lessons learned in the institutional scandals of the 1960s have been forgotten.

A CASE STUDY OF CHANGE

Any management textbook states what needs to be done in these services: how they should define clearly the most important goals they will work towards, how they should provide the support staff will need to achieve them and how they should monitor progress and ensure compliance. There is already an impressive body of research, largely American, which demonstrates how these things might be done. Studies address what staff should be trained in (e.g. Thousand *et al.*, 1986), how they might be best trained (Anderson, 1987), how they can be directed and motivated to work well (e.g. Reid *et al.*, 1989) and so on.

In one of these three services we have tried to help managers address these issues using this store of knowledge. A major problem for this service had been increasing and unpredictable placement breakdowns. Our view was that these occurred because throughout the service there was insufficient skill in working constructively with service users. The intervention adopted took as its initial focus the model of care provided in all of the houses. The aim was to improve the quality of care in each house, by replacing 'minding' with skilled support to facilitate the involvement and independence of service users, and thereby to increase the resilience of the whole service and reduce the likelihood of placement breakdowns. This 'active support' model of care was derived from the work described above.

Often there are major obstacles to providing this model of care because services are poorly designed (too institutional) or under-resourced (too few staff). In this case, all the houses met minimum criteria for introducing the model: the resources were available but were not being effectively used.

The introduction of the new model of care was organized as a 'whole environment training' intervention (Whiffen, 1984; Mansell, 1988a), in which 12 days' hands-on training was given to each staff team in working with the people they served. The researchers took the lead in designing this training and in delivering it to the first eight houses, although training was jointly provided with the middle managers of the service in order to strengthen their competence and role in providing practice leadership. A second group of eight houses received training from managers with support and advice from the researchers as consultants and then managers took responsibility for completing the training in all houses in the service.

This approach was chosen because practical training has consistently been shown to be superior to classroom training in producing changed performance on the job (Anderson, 1987); training in situ should increase the likelihood of maintenance and generalization; and supporting managers to do the training rather than using external trainers exclusively was intended to strengthen the managers' role in providing leadership in quality of care and their ownership of the intervention.

In addition there were many administrative changes to emphasize the importance of active support by care staff and leadership in quality of care by first-line and middle managers; a series of orientation workshops on issues such as challenging behaviour, communication skills and teaching; and sending four key care staff on a university diploma course in working with people who have challenging behaviour, two staff on a Trainers' Development Programme and one trainer on an MA programme in learning disability.

The third component of the intervention to improve services was improvement in information about the quality of service received by clients and those features of the service's organization which were most directly related to quality. The aim here was to correct the imbalance in management information that existed because there was so much less information about quality than finance or personnel, and to increase the extent to which management decisions were evaluated against their impact on quality.

Finally the service reviewed how it managed crises which did occur. The aim here was to develop a process for predicting which services were most vulnerable, for gathering the resources necessary to help people manage through a difficult period and for avoiding emergency transfers to institutional care. The products were written procedures for use within the service and initiatives to explain clearly what the service wanted from the two other agencies most involved when crises did occur – the mental health services and the police.

The impact of this intervention was immediate. Whole environment training allowed dramatic improvements to be made in the houses with existing resources. Many service users were assisted to participate in everyday activities for the first time since their move to the service. In seven of the eight houses where whole-environment training was first carried out, the trainers' report indicated greater levels of involvement in a wider range of activities by service users. Staff became more skilled at sharing activities and responded enthusiastically to the extra help they were getting. For some of the house managers, the clear priority given to achieving client outcomes and the leadership role taken by their own managers made them more confident in asking for help.

One result of the training was a marked shift in reputation for a small but significant number of individuals with special needs. For example, a deaf and blind client in one house with whom staff had been at a loss to know how to work was, by the end of the training period, being helped to prepare meals. In another house a person with severe self-injury defeated most attempts by staff to involve her in any activity. The training helped introduce a number of reactive management strategies to enable staff to work through difficult situations and also a 'positive programming' inter-vention which made the young woman's environment more predictable and understandable to her through the presentation of similar requests and activities at pre-arranged times. The outcome of this was that for the first time, staff could interact with her in such a way that she would not injure herself. This allowed her to go out shopping and to cafés, activities she particularly enjoyed, as well as participate in everyday activities around the house.

These individual examples challenged any complacency about previously acceptable levels of staff and managers' performance and achieved recognition in the service as they happened, producing optimism and enthusiasm in the service's managers.

The number of people in the service who took part in the whole-environment training steadily increased, as did the number of houses defined by managers as meeting a set of basic criteria. The service was able to cease making out-of-area placements. The last four people who were transferred out-of-area were brought back to local services. Within-agency transfers continue, so it is too soon to say that the competence of services has increased enough to avoid placement breakdowns. Rather, what seems to have happened is that changed perceptions by managers and staff have made them take different decisions in advance of sufficiently improved front-line staff performance. Managers of the service say that the knowledge that there is a workable alternative to the 'minding' model of care, coupled with the evidence of what was achieved in the whole-environment training, has made them determined to develop better services and not necessarily to respond to crises by seeking out-of-area placements.

In terms of the outcomes experienced by clients, however, there were mixed results. There was an increase in community contacts, but the service's own observational data on levels of client engagement and staff–client contact is very patchy. What information there is suggests rising levels of engagement in meaningful activity and staff contact over the first ten months, followed by a decline and some evidence of increases again. However, information collected independently by the researchers on two occasions since the initial evaluation showed no change in these areas. The implication of this must be that the achievements of the whole-environment training have not been maintained.

In attributing the changes that have occurred in the performance of this service to particular interventions it is important to recognize that the project took place against a background of wider change. There have been some new senior and middle managers and increased staff turnover, which have probably helped the process of change as people who were not prepared to take part left the organization. Less helpful changes have been cuts in staffing as the service has borne a share of National Health Service (NHS) underfunding and the uncertainty generated by the reorganization of health and social services following the 1989 NHS and Community Care Act. The extent to which managers have been able to maintain a clear focus on quality has reflected the relative lack of priority given by their superiors to improving quality compared with attending to the competing demands of reorganization. Finally, the unbending bureaucracy of large organizations has also played its part: compared with the kind of employment practice which underpins much American work on staff performance, these managers faced very time-consuming and difficult procedures to deal with middle managers or staff who failed to improve their performance, and extremely limited opportunities for differentially rewarding and supporting good work. Eventually, this service was split up between several statutory and voluntary organizations in line with the community care reforms.

THE LIMITS OF INFLUENCE

Despite some improvements, then, this intervention did not successfully tackle the problem of low engagement in staffed housing. In one sense this can simply be put down to poor maintenance of trained performance in the light of failure to implement effective monitoring. The interesting question is why it should be so difficult, given the published research, to put these things into practice?

In these concluding comments, I want to speculate about the answer to this question. Firstly, it seems plausible that cross-cultural transfer of interventions is complicated by the researcher's definition of what the intervention does and does not include. For example, American research usually assumes a managerial framework in which compliance with management instructions is required and where there can be quick and certain penalties for non-compliance. British culture, at least, is not like this; staff do not seem to start with the assumption that they should do what their managers want. This is not simply a question of unionization – community services are much less unionized than institutions. Instead it might reflect staff's (accurate) perception that their managers know less about the job than they do, or at least are less skilled at doing it; or that the penalties of establishing a precedent for easy compliance in one area are exploitation in others. Thus sceptical, defensive staff may resist and undermine the introduction of new ways of working not because they object strongly to them but because they open up the possibility of being held accountable for problems caused by poorly thought-out management plans or of opening themselves to worse conditions later.

Related to this is the observation that, in practice, senior managers are apparently indifferent to the quality of care in these services. In the case study, the managers of the learning disability service were committed to achieving quality but the generic health authority managers to whom they were accountable made only budgetary demands. Perhaps the best practical illustration of this is that at the end of our work the government reorganized services to introduce a split between the 'purchasers' of services and the 'providers'. Part of the rationale for this was to strengthen monitoring and accountability. The service proposed to the new purchasing agency that they should be held accountable for a range of quality goals including levels of engagement in meaningful activity. The purchasing body explicitly removed these detailed requirements as not required; apparently on the grounds that since they did not require such detailed evidence for other client groups it would not be appropriate to do so in learning disability.

Management commitment in North American services seems to have been fuelled partly by the specialist organization of services and partly by legal challenges and the mandating of individual habilitation planning. Braddock *et al.* (1995) suggests that a background of civil rights work in local politics may also predict commitment to community services and in the Scandinavian countries, as well as clear legal frameworks, there has been a strong tradition of partnership between parents, users and service agencies. In Britain, in contrast, the movement for community services has been dominated by professionals and alliances with users and parents are weak; services are embedded in generic organizations facing many other pressing demands and there is no enforceable right to a certain quality of service.

Thus, in a sense, the staff and managers of the service in the case study may have been accurately reading their employers' real priorities.

REFORMULATING THE AGENDA FOR SOCIAL ACTION

In this case, what might be done to improve the prospects for the development of community services which are of good quality? Despite any desire by government to turn away from the problems of services for people with learning disabilities there continues to be as much scope for public concern about standards in community services as there was in institutions. The pressure for action is therefore likely to continue. In these circumstances it will be important for research to continue to correctly attribute the reasons for those problems – for example, to focus on management weakness rather than blaming clients as beyond hope.

Secondly, there is unfinished business in the building of a more powerful coalition in favour of community services in Britain. Professional, user and parent interests are fragmented and sometimes divided in their public position on community care. A clearer message will be needed before government, or at least the decision-makers for the agencies concerned, feel compelled to improve services.

Deinstitutionalization in the Norwegian welfare state 5

Jan Tøssebro

Three decades ago, two major problems confronted the Norwegian service system for people with mental retardation: institutions were too small and beds were too few (St. prp. 36 (parliamentary bill), 1960–61). The total number of beds fell considerably short of needs, and according to prevailing knowledge, a mean number of 50 residents per institution (153 in central institutions and 25 in others) was definitely suboptimal.

Since then, a major shift in attitudes has taken place. In Norway, all long-stay mental retardation institutions are supposed to be closed during the first half of the 1990s. This policy was promoted by a very critical official committee report (NOU, 1985:34), stating, for example, that: 'the living conditions for people with mental retardation in institutions are humanly, socially and culturally unacceptable' (p.12) and that 'the situation cannot be substantially changed by reorganising work or increasing resource supply' (p.25). Similar descriptions can be found in the international research literature, the most prominent probably still being that by Goffman (1961). In general, however, research findings on institutional care are more ambiguous, and frequently consistent with the statement by Zigler *et al.* (1986) that 'as in earlier research, institutional variables were not predictive of the behaviours examined' (p.10). In 1990 the same first author recommends less attention to normalization and deinstitutionalization, and more to 'bettering the lives of retarded individuals' (Zigler *et al.*, 1990, p.1).

These contradictory opinions may reflect many things, but most likely they reflect different points of departure. There are numerous ways to classify approaches to the study of institutions. Gustavsson and Söder (1990) discuss the civil rights v. social science perspectives and Bruininks (1990), in a comment on Zigler *et al.* (1990), argues that policy-oriented research may yield different results from that driven by a purely academic orientation. For the purposes of this Chapter four approaches are of interest.

The first has a social policy orientation. It is descriptive and could be called the 'univariate' scandal model. The residential institutions are regarded as a part of the redistributive system – as a social policy response to the needs of a group of citizens. Consequently, the institutions should be evaluated as a social policy, and the key question is whether services are good enough according to current national social policy standards. Descriptions according to such a perspective are frequently in keeping with the Norwegian official committee report (NOU, 1985:34), though the recommendations could equally well simply be for 'more money'.

The next approach could be characterized by the analysis of variance. The main question is whether institutional variables, or the institutions as a specific organizational species, can explain the outcomes. This does not mean a proper causal analysis. Occasions where data (and ethics) would permit this are rare, partly because 'institution' is not well defined as a variable, and partly because people are unlikely to be randomly assigned to residential settings (Lieberson, 1985; Butterfield, 1987; Landesman and Butterfield, 1987). Studies of this type include a wide range of dependent and independent variables, and as noted by Zigler *et al.* (1986), such research frequently shows that 'institutional variables were not predictive', but more often that 'effects ... are complex and multiple determined' (Zigler *et al.*, 1990, p.10). According to Gustavsson and Söder (1990), the general finding in this research is that the result 'all depends'. Although divergent findings definitely exist (for example, Felce *et al.*, 1991; Raynes *et al.*, 1987), the analysis of variance tends to dissolve the scandal.

Research based on the third point of departure involves 'outward bound' studies (Booth *et al.*, 1990) and is generally optimistic concerning the effects of deinstitutionalization (Larson and Lakin, 1989; Conroy and Bradley, 1985; Chapters 10 and 11). Certainly, some residents are reinstitutionalized, frequently due to behaviour problems (Sutter *et al.*, 1980; Intagliata and Willer, 1982; Vitello *et al.*, 1983), and reports on social network and activity pattern are ambiguous. However, the residents themselves seem to prefer the new services (Birenbaum and Re, 1979; Schalock and Lilley, 1986; Edgerton *et al.*, 1984), and Swedish research tends to report more consistently favourable outcomes than literature in the English language (Sonnander and Nilsson-Embro, 1984; Ericsson *et al.*, 1987; Thorsell, 1989). Scepticism concerning inappropriate design for causal inferences, however, also applies for this approach.

The last approach is similar to French structuralism: the institutions are regarded as surface phenomena, while the basic problem is some kind of underlying force or generator. Wolfensberger's (1972; 1992) account of the process of devaluation illustrates this, at least when discussing problems of new services. The reasoning of Foucault (1961), Scull (1977) and Cohen (1985) could also be classified here. These studies tend to be ambitious, almost world-historic in design, and the policy message is important: if you do nothing about the 'generator', reforms tend to be superficial and the problems are likely to reappear under a new guise.

The main part of this chapter is guided by the social policy perspective, and discusses the dismantling of residential institutions for people with mental retardation in Norway. The question is whether institutional life did meet the social policy standards. Later in the chapter, however, the same facts are discussed from other perspectives to address the question of whether is it possible to attribute the problems of institutional life to institutional variables. It is important to pay attention to the possibility that institutions are scapegoats, because if so, dismantling them is less likely to bring about the real changes desired.

First, a brief outline of the institution-based system and its history in Norway is required. A detailed description is available in Tøssebro (1992).

A HISTORICAL OUTLINE

Residential institutions for people with mental retardation are a rather recent phenomenon in Norway. The first 'home' was established in 1898, but until 1950 very few people were served. Roughly speaking, the growth period was the 1950s and 1960s (Figure 5.1), considerably later than other countries (Chapter 1 as comparative data). From the early 1970s there have only been minor changes in the number of people served. The institutionalized population, about 5500 in the 1970s, corresponds roughly to 0.14% of the Norwegian population (the same figure as in the United States in the 1980s (Bruininks et al., 1987)), and includes about a third of the people administratively classified as people with mental retardation (about half of the adults).

In the 1950s and 1960s most facilities were private, though financially supported by public authorities. In 1969 full responsibility was placed on county authorities. Independently, but at about the same time, a policy change took place. Scandals occurred, words like segregation assumed negative connotations, and the parental society was established in 1967. However, contrary to some other countries, the shift was not yet a dein-stitutionalization movement – except for the children who gradually disappeared from institutions. The key words were 'decentralization' and 'improved living conditions', and this actually happened (Table 5.1). A number of new small institutions were established, and the number of residents were reduced in existing institutions. During the 1980s, the

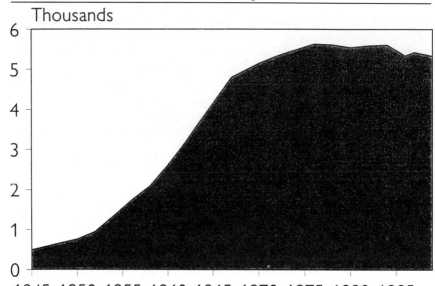

Figure 5.1 People in mental retardation institutions in Norway 1945–89.

institutions reached what Norwegians like to think of as high quality in international comparison.

In other countries, the new small facilities (usually 5–15 residents) would probably be called group homes, thus illustrating that the definition of institutions varies. In Norway, the definition is juridical: an institution is licensed and run according to the law on hospitals. This implies, however, that working and living is subject to a medical or problem rationale rather than a living or housing rationale.

EXPANDING THE WELFARE STATE

The improvement in the 1970s did not silence the criticisms. The parental society put total dismantling of institutional care on the political agenda around 1980, and this became public policy in 1988 (planning period 1988–90, implementation period 1991–95). Ideological keywords were 'a society for all' and 'citizen rights'. It was also argued that 'it is time the welfare state includes everyone'. This can be read as requesting generic services, but also that the living conditions should meet current social policy standards. These standards are rarely strict written requirements, but rather a tacit assessment incorporated in the concept – or ambition – of the welfare state.

One aspect of the welfare state is the responsibility for securing basic

Table 5.1 Changes from 1971–89 in residential institutions for mentally retarded persons in Norway

	1971	1989
Staff per resident (1970 and 1988)	0.63	1.78
Mean no. of residents per:		
central institution	228.00	142.00
other institution	25.00	13.00
living unit	22.90	6.50
sleeping room	2.60	1.00
% of residents in central institution	65.00	45.00
Mean square metre per resident (sleeping room excl.)	3.34	18.67

needs for the citizens. Such a definition is, however, much too loose (Esping-Andersen, 1990). It is actually consistent, for example, with the British Poor Laws of 1834, a system based on the principle that getting support should be so unpleasant that only people in desperate need would apply (the 'less eligibility' principle). Discouragement was the rationale, the aspect of social control and punishment were considerable, and support was intended to be stigmatizing.

Another aspect of the welfare state is conceptualized in Titmuss's (1974) famous distinction between the residual and institutional redistributive welfare models. These models could be seen as a description of a continuum: the British Poor Laws of 1834 as the residual extreme, and total emancipation from the labour market – the classical 'to each according to his needs' – as the other extreme. The ambition of the welfare state is not to disregard the labour market. The value base is more like a compromise between 'to each according to their performance' and 'to each according to their needs' (cf. Martinussen, 1988). The definition of the welfare state would, simplistically, be that services and support are taken for granted as citizen rights, and should be generous enough to sustain decent living conditions. Decency, rather than discouragement, is the guiding principle.

The expansion of the welfare state to include people with mental retardation was to introduce a new quality standard. Services are supposed to provide living conditions that are not just 'good enough for people with mental retardation', but would pass as decent for other citizens as well.

RESIDENTIAL INSTITUTIONS AS SOCIAL POLICY

Did residential institutions for Norwegians with mental retardation meet contemporary social policy standards? The discussion is confined to two examples, housing and activity, and is based on data from three Norwegian counties (N=591, cf. Tøssebro, 1990).

Housing standards show considerable variation. Some are old houses, physically organized around a corridor, just like an old-fashioned nursing home but, by and large, most seem to be of an acceptable standard. The houses are reasonably modern and well-equipped, just like any other house on all but one measure: they are crowded.

The housing conditions can be compared to those of a child of an average middle-class family, with a single semi-private room and some rooms available to all. In Norway, when these arrangements apply to adults living apart from their family they meet the official definition of overcrowding. The written standards are somewhat obscure on group living but approximately 90% of the residents are overcrowded by the criteria of the Central Bureau of Statistics, and most of the houses (at least 75%) would not obtain loans in the Norwegian National Housing Bank because space per person is below the requirement of decent housing.

However, the problems that do not reveal themselves in statistics are even more important. This concerns the interpretation or meaning of housing: a house or flat is more than just a place to stay. From an ethological perspective it is the core private territory, and in the semiotic perspective, it is a presentation of self. The territorial problem is illustrated by sayings like 'my house is my castle'. The house marks off a certain area where private life is expected to be protected. Others have no entrance unless invited. In normal everyday life the territorial dimension is an obvious regulator of interaction. It is a 'taken-for-granted' that we do not think much about, except when it is violated.

The territoriality of residents in Norwegian institutions is violated because (see Table 5.2):

- People are located and relocated according to administrative rationale rather than their own choice.
- Markers of private space are absent (for example, names are rarely present on the door plate, few people have a key to their private room,

there are communal rooms from which the resident is excluded, some people own nothing except a cassette tape recorder).
- Residents have little influence on important decisions affecting their everyday life.
- The other people in the house (staff and fellow residents) are neither chosen nor family.

Almost no-one participates in decisions concerning whom to live with, and only about a third of the residents are said to get on well with their peers. If staff assessments are correct, no more than 18% have a close relationship with fellow residents.

Substantial variation exists among people and living units, particularly regarding markers of private space, influence in everyday life, and how well people interact with their fellow residents. In general, however, it is an accurate description to say that people's territory is invaded – and this territory is crowded.

From a semiotic perspective, an institution is a linguistic sign. The building tells a tacit story – a presentation of images, so important to the Wolfensberger (1972) tradition. Whether we like it or not, the general public see the larger institutions as symbols of devaluation and exclusion – with a little dash of danger. This was perfectly illustrated by a man who had recently left a central institution in Norway: when he left, he took some of the furniture from his former living unit. As it turned out, he did not want it, and made staff advertise it for sale. A man responded, and bought it all. As soon as the buyer left the house, the resident roared with laughter, saying: 'That guy was a real fool. I wonder what he would say, if he ever knew that the furniture had been at the institution for 15 years.'

Nearly all the houses, even among the small institutions, did carry symbols of difference. As an interviewer reported: 'Staff frequently said the house is just like any house, but – as soon as I found the neighbourhood, I didn't have any problem picking the right house'.

The second example is activity. Mental retardation institutions are frequently criticized for inactivity but, generally speaking, reported participation in leisure activities in Norwegian institutions actually seems to be about the same as the rest of the population, and 96% are engaged in some kind of daytime activity: sheltered work, education or day-centre activities (Table 5.3). These figures, however, obscure the fact that a substantial proportion participate in very few activities, while a minority (15–20%) show an activity pattern comparable to adolescents. For example, 60% of people have daytime activities which occupy less than 20 hours a week, and 40% less than 10 hours (Table 5.4). The 'missing' daytime occupation is not compensated by leisure activities. Those 'working'

Table 5.2 Indicators of 'territorial invasion'

A. Missing markers of territory	
	%
Name not on the doorplate	89
Rooms exist to which the resident has no entrance	72

B. Authority over territory	
	%
Participates in decisions concerning[a]:	
relocation	22
whom to live with	5
meals	41
clothing	66
furniture	30
'Some' autonomy according to general staff evaluation[b]	15

[a] Respondents have replied 'decides him-/herself' or 'participates'.
[b] Staff are asked to assess 'influence in everyday life' on a five point scale. Top score (1) is 'autonomy about the same as me', and bottom (5) 'none at all'. Responses 1 and 2 are included here.

C. Relations to persons on territory	
	%
Close relation to one fellow resident	18
Fellow residents suit each other	31
Socializes with fellow residents[c]	54

[c] The percentage spending at least 'some' leisure time with fellow residents. Mere co-presence at the same time and place is excluded.

few hours also participate in few leisure activities (Pearson's r varies from 0.24–0.36 on different indicators (Tøssebro, 1992)). A rough estimate is that 35% live clearly inactive lives, while another 20% come close to such a description.

Activities also call for interpretation and the most important activity in our culture is work. There are many reasons for the pre-eminent position of work, among which are that work is a most important source of independence. There is more to this than achieving financial independence through earning money: participation in production proves personal

Table 5.3 Primary occupation

	%
Sheltered employment – ordinary site	4
Sheltered employment – special site	14
Vocational training	2
Day centre – 'work activity'	22
Day centre – non-work activity	26
Education	28
No occupation	4
Total	100
N	591

Table 5.4 Hours per week in primary and secondary occupation

	%
1–10 hours	42
11–19 hours	17
20–25 hours	16
26–35 hours	19
more than 35 hours	5
Total	99
N	591

worth and usefulness, and as such, work is a part of the construction of the full and independent citizen. Norwegian culture is some kind of secularized Calvinism: people show their worth through achievement – preferably at work.

This argument is obviously somewhat crude. It is, however, important to note since the work of people with mental retardation is usually framed by arrangements which tell us that it is not real work. It goes on out of place, and the pay is symbolic both in that average pay levels are extremely low and that it signifies that the work is pretend. It does not tell that 'you are doing a useful job', but rather that 'we are nice people who give you some occupation'. Pretend work is likely to be preferred to inactivity or leisure activities all day, though some residents of institutions and other disabled people refuse to work if they think it is a pretence. The point is that the activity is not work as a source of independence: it is rather an integrated part of the individual's dependence.

In summary, this means that institutional life falls considerably short of prevailing social policy standards. This is so using traditional criteria like overcrowding and under-employment (or income and possessions). However, even more important are some taken-for-granted qualities of everyday life: the symbolism of housing and the invasion of privacy, and the pretend qualities of work (though the value compromise of the welfare state makes work more difficult to interpret).

THE IMPACT OF INSTITUTIONAL VARIABLES

It is tempting to attribute causality to the description above, and the decision to dismantle the institutions in Norway actually implied such attribution. The official committee did regard the poor conditions as a product of institutional care, and considered improvement unlikely to be successful.

On the other hand, as already noted, studies of institutions frequently show that institutional variables are not predictive or that results depend on other factors. In general, multivariate analyses of Norwegian data (cf. Tøssebro, 1992a) repeat such findings. This may obviously be because all subjects are living in institutions. It would, however, be premature to disregard the fact that facility sizes vary from 4–192 (thus including what is internationally known as group homes), and that most indicators on living conditions show a considerable variance. This variance, however, is rarely explained by institutional variables (institution size, living unit size, location, etc). Crudely, the most important independent variable is the skills of the resident. However, some variation is not explained at all: for example, the value of R Square (the proportion of variation in the dependent variable explained by the model) is just 0.11 for 'having friends (fellow residents excluded)' by skills, institution size, living unit size and age. Alternatively, some findings are simply explained: frequency of contact with parents is strongly correlated with physical distance to the parents' home and slightly correlated to the parents' age – both indicating the importance of practical problems.

A wide range of living condition variables are correlated with the residents' adaptive behaviour, for example, income, possessions, relationship with fellow residents, indicators of territorial invasion, activity, etc. In all these examples, the standardized regression coefficient exceeds 0.40, controlled for institution size, living unit size, age, sex, county and years since admission. The findings may have two explanations: firstly, the poor conditions may reflect realities of the impairment, for example, if a person cannot express themselves, participation in decisions about everyday life is not exactly straightforward; and secondly, the institutions may give priority to people with mild mental retardation. Both explanations are likely to be true. It is, for example, disquieting to make the two minute walk – at the same central institution – from a low priority ward for people with profound mental retardation, to high priority units populated by less handicapped individuals.

There are, however, exceptions to the 'disappointing' minor importance of institutional variables. Living unit size is correlated with overcrowding, though this is almost by definition, but also with territorial invasion. This is at first sight not in keeping with the bulk of earlier research (King et al., 1971; McCormick et al., 1975; Zigler and Balla 1977; Landesman-Dwyer et al., 1980; Landesman-Dwyer, 1981), which has played down the effect of size, though divergent findings do exist. The difference arises, however, because earlier research has not paid sufficient attention to really small units. The data show an asymptotic relationship, and the impact of unit size is substantial in the below five residents' size range (Tøssebro, 1991). This result is in accordance with research on small group interaction, and what Grunewald (1992) calls 'the principle of the small group': each person should know the others well enough to predict reactions to approaches.

Before ending this section, it is appropriate to comment upon two issues that do not arise from multivariate analysis, but from alternative explanations of poor living conditions. Both indicate the same conclusions as the above analyses: that problem generators are to be found elsewhere and are not limited to the particular organizational species called institutions.

The first alternative explanation is simply that the real problem is shortage of resources; a matter of political priorities. This can for example probably explain both overcrowding and the existence of large (and less private) wards. The post-1970 history shows that as funding increased, reduction of unit size, overcrowding and institution size had a high priority inside the institutional system. There is no reason to believe that this would not continue if more resources were added. Another example is provided by the inactivity of the less skilled residents. According to experienced staff it was perfectly possible to construct a more active existence.

The main obstacle was, however, not organization but resources. The second alternative explanation is that problems are generated by regulations that are not restricted to institutions. This, for example, concerns the pretend character of work. The regulations that make work a pretence apply to all kinds of sheltered employment – inside as well as outside institutions – and there is no reason to expect that deinstitutionalization changes this. Thus, it may be argued that the Norwegian welfare state violates the guiding principle of decency in this matter. This violation is partly due to the difficulties in setting up a system of pay for non- or low-productive work that is on the one hand decent, but at the same time does not violate the 'to each according to their performance' part of the welfare state compromise.

BUT DOES DEINSTITUTIONALIZATION MAKE A DIFFERENCE?

The research described above does not indicate dramatic effects of organizational change. On the other hand, the 'outward bound' studies usually show improvements, and there are a lot of encouraging things happening in Norway as well: expenditure has increased by about 50% from 1989–1992 (but no increase from 1992–93); houses are better, less crowded, less physically segregated, and less deviant; and more people (but far from all) are served. Research on the new homes show a substantial change in staff behaviour, particularly concerning private territory (Jensen, 1992). Symbols of personal space and privacy are likely to emerge, along with personal possessions and a 'pretend visitor' interaction style from staff. This is indeed encouraging, although there is still a long way to go.

Does this mean that 'the analysis of variance' approach misses important mechanisms, or is it possible that the positive impact of deinstitutionalization is not an effect of the organizational change at all, but rather some kind of Hawthorne effect? Maybe the change in itself is the most important generator of improvement because it attracts political attention and triggers a professional discourse.

Political attention does not just mean that services for people with mental retardation are on the agenda, but also that the lifestyle and living conditions have to be defended by arguments. Today, such defence is unlikely to be legitimate unless based on current social political standards.

The most important change is consequently a change in what could pass as a legitimate argument, and this did temporarily undermine the traditional budgetary argument – that 'this is too expensive'.

Dismantling institutions also goes with a professional discourse; a re-examination of practice. This occurs at a time when organizational change facilitates a breakdown of habitual routines. The new routines are subjected to discursive requirements: verbalization and defence according to current ideologies. One aspect of this is conceptual – an institution is not just a place, it is some kind of mental category that affects perceptions and interaction rules. In Norway, the concept of institution seems to favour attitudes fit for a medical or problem rationale. In someone else's home, people are expected and likely to behave according to a different set of interaction rules, and if the residential facility is conceptualized as a home both staff and local government are likely to be more aware of the territorial problems (although, as Jensen (1992) notes, too much respect for territoriality can also lead to neglect).

This kind of reasoning calls for some kind of 'what was first' discussion: the deinstitutionalization process or the activation of the value base of the welfare state. Deinstitutionalization was clearly a part of a larger improvement movement already present; the expansion of the welfare state. And the deinstitutionalization must be evaluated as a part of such a movement, rather than an organizational experiment. But on the other hand, it has stimulated both political attention and professional discourse. The larger movement has been reinforced by deinstitutionalization, and more money has been forthcoming. It is, however, important to notice that this kind of mechanism depends upon levels of attention which may not be likely to last for long.

Does this end in some conclusion? More like a warning. It is premature to disregard the problems of attributing causality to institutional variables, and it is important to be cautious not to expect too much from organizational change in itself. Deinstitutionalization is, however, important as an integrated part of the improvement movement. This is maybe best illustrated by the semiotics of residential institutions. It is frequently reported, actually as early as by Edgerton (1967), that one important aspect of deinstitutionalization is the experience of leaving a place which signifies social devaluation: Goffman (1961) describes the reverse process happening in admission. But it is premature to regard institutions as the cause of their signification. Mental retardation is stigmatized in itself, and it is very optimistic to believe that this will change as the institutions close. On the other hand, it is a classical sociological and anthropological argument – in the tradition of Durkheim (1915) – that materialization has a certain impact in itself. The flag and national anthem reflect attitudes, but at the same time they evoke and reinforce the very same attitudes in the same way, institutions reflect, evoke and reinforce devaluation. It is necessary to shut down such symbols, though it is equally important to be aware of the possibility that the new nursery-like houses could assume the same signification some years ahead.

PART TWO:
Models of
Community Services

Housing for the person with intellectual handicap   6

Kent Ericsson

In Sweden, as in most countries in Western Europe, it was during the second half of the nineteenth century that organized provision was made specifically for people dependent on help and support from others. Increased industrialization and urbanization put new demands on the citizen. In Sweden, one such demand, significant and consequential for people with intellectual handicap, was the introduction of compulsory schooling. In pace with the establishment of the ordinary school system, special school institutions were started for those who could not cope with the demands of the ordinary schools. These became the first forms of state support for this group of handicapped people. When demands on achievement increased in these schools, two additional institutional forms were developed, asylums for those with extensive needs and occupational-homes for those who left school on reaching adulthood. The 'educable' were provided with education at the school institutions, and work was provided at the occupational-home. The 'ineducable' were referred to a life at an asylum, living in simple conditions, irrespective of whether they were children, adolescents, adults or elderly. Through this process the Swedish institutional tradition was established. It was further reinforced by legislation, which in the mid-1950s closely regulated how society was to provide support for this group. But as their roots were in the pedagogical tradition, Swedish institutions remained comparatively small (Söder, 1978).

THE COMMUNITY SERVICE TRADITION

The change from institutional to community services, provided through housing, employment and a life in the community, has its roots in the welfare society as it was established during the mid-1940s. More modern social services had to be developed if the idea of a welfare society for the public was to be realized. The creation of these services gave rise to new means of providing support to people with handicaps. Parallel to institutional services, society could use modern social services and thereby had two ways of channelling its support to people with handicaps (Ericsson, 1985b; Ericsson, 1986b; Ericsson, 1987a).

As a result of the debate on the nature of the support of society which took place at the beginning of the 1940s, the Committee for the Partially Able-bodied was given the task of identifying suitable forms of support for people with handicaps, so that they could experience a good life. The Committee was critical of many aspects of the care being provided for the partially able-bodied in residential institutions. It noted that responsibility was only being taken for those already cared for in the institution while no concern was given to preventative health work. The Committee criticized the coercive system represented by the institutions and the patriarchal view which characterized attitudes to people with handicaps (SOU, 1946:24).

On the basis of their criticism of institutional care, and a vision of new opportunities for services in a welfare society, the view of the Committee was that the partially able-bodied should also have a right to services being established within the framework of the welfare society.

> ... a given principle, that the partially able-bodied should, as far as possible, be included in the ordinary system of social services, which is under development in our country.
>
> (SOU, 1946:24, p.28)

In order to realize this it was considered important that the support of society be built in such a way that it be available for all.

> The institutions of society must be adjusted so as to justly, and preferably in context, include all individuals, irrespective of whichever category they belong .
>
> (SOU, 1946:24, p.28)

It was believed that this would have positive consequences for the people concerned.

> Psychologically 'normalisation' of living conditions, education, employment support etc for partially able-bodied people, is surely a great advantage.
>
> (SOU, 1946:24, p.28)

That the welfare society should also take responsibility for people with handicaps was, according to the Committee, an expression of:

... a basic civic demand: it is in entire accordance with the essence of our democratic concept, that equal human values and their equal rights be placed in the foreground.

(SOU, 1946:24, p.28)

In these quotations a socio-political idea was expressed which was termed the normalization principle (Kommittén för partiellt arbetsföra, 1949):

'The normalization principle', as prescribed by the committee, proposes, amongst other things, that special institutions for the partially able-bodied, for education, training, etc should be the exception, not the rule.

(Kommittén för partiellt arbetsföra, 1949)

This implied that a stand was taken for the normalization of the conditions of life for people with handicaps, a policy which should be pursued as an alternative to living a life separated from the lives of those without handicaps. The means of achieving this was through the development of modern social services, within the framework of the welfare society, which were accessible to all people. This should be seen in the context of the socio-political ideas formulated in the mid-1940s, at the end of the Second World War, in a period of democratic and economic optimism.

The Committee did not refer to any special group among the partially able-bodied but included all people with handicaps, even the 'feeble-minded', the expression used for people with intellectual handicap. This idea, however, only applied to those with a mild handicap, who, as a consequence of receiving support could increase their productive ability and thereby their ability to support themselves. The policy of the Committee did not include those with a more severe handicap, those termed 'unfit for work'. They were instead referred to 'modernized institutional care' that is to say, to a continuation of the institutional system.

THE NORMALIZATION PROCESS

With the recognition of the normalization principle a new socio-political direction on how society should support people with handicaps was established. This had consequences for the nature of the societal support that developed during the following years. With regard to provisions for people with intellectual handicap these have, through a series of legislative measures, swung from a traditional institutional form of support to a broader and more integrated system of services. According to the 1985 Act the large institutions are no longer recognized as a means of providing support, instead the right to a life in the ordinary community is acknowledged even for adults with extensive support needs. From the 1946 understanding of the normalization principle, which was the first step away from the institutional tradition, it has taken 40 years before all those with intellectual handicap have been included.

This also puts into perspective present-day community services. Considering that they have their roots in the normalization principle of 1946 the first assertion is that the change has been going on for a long period. The development of community services for all has taken place during a 50-year period, parallel with the dissolution of the institutional tradition, and the task is still going on.

In this normalization principle there is also a societal framework for the emergence of community services. It was during the years after the Second World War that the community tradition – the move away from the institutional system – was developed. These were years of democratic optimism, the beginning of a period of economic prosperity, with far-reaching structural change in society.

This process of normalization can be found at several levels. At an individual level this development has meant a switch from an institutional life to an increased participation in the life of the local community, where the person lives together with people without handicap. This community participation has also affected others. For relatives this has meant that the son or daughter no longer has to be visited at a residential institution, but in a house in the local community. Neighbours, and those providing services locally are, to an increasing extent, coming into contact with people with intellectual handicap.

At an organizational level changes have occurred in the forms of service provided. A development of services has taken place which contributes to the participation of people in community life. Teaching is being provided in the community school, where children without handicaps attend. New forms of service have also developed for adults, which enables them to be in places and environments where other adults spend their time. Group homes have made it possible to provide housing in ordinary housing areas, and daily activities are now organized so that activities for these people can take place together with those without handicaps.

Parallel to this development is the dissolution of institutional forms of care. Forms of care which do not promote, or which hinder participation in community life, for example, special hospitals, children's homes and boarding schools, are being closed down. Even the new forms of community services are going through a process of change, for example, day activity centres which do not contribute adequately to community participation, are undergoing change and development (Ericsson, 1981; Ericsson, 1990).

Another change found within this normalization process concerns the way society perceives people with intellectual handicap. The institutional tradition, with two types of establishments – the school institution and the asylum – reflected two ways of regarding these people. Those with a mild handicap who were considered 'educable' were provided with schooling and were termed as 'pupils', while those with a more severe handicap, who were referred to asylums and residential homes – the 'ineducable' – were seen as 'patients' in need of care.

Thus the perspective used has implications for the social role ascribed to people with intellectual handicap, and this was the basis on which community services were built. In speaking of a democratic right to a life outside the institution, the view being expressed is of the individual as a full citizen.

The social role of a citizen can therefore be said to be that which is associated with community services and the development of this type of support is a logical consequence of this perspective. From these different social roles within institutional and community services, one can see also a change at societal level within this normalization process. This change comprises the shift caused by leaving the perception of these persons as 'pupils' or 'patients', to the development of a perspective regarding them as 'citizens'.

THE NEED FOR HOUSING

Housing has a basic function in the life of a person. The characteristics of their house and the life they live there, both inside and outside, contribute to the quality of the life they can experience. There is not, however, a clear answer to the question of housing for people with intellectual handicap. Whereas some maintain that special institutions are suitable for them, others consider that they should have the opportunity to live in ordinary housing.

When Swedish society began to establish its support for people with intellectual handicap during the nineteenth century, it was located in residential institutions of various kinds. The only form of support outside the institution was a type of family-care which provided housing, most often in farming areas, but which was used only to a limited extent (Söder, 1978). In the event of a lack of other means of support, those in need had to live on their own or in a family.

During the 1940s plans were initiated for the shift from institutional care, a change which led to new forms of housing outside the institution. The 1954 Act introduced the concept of 'open-care', expressing the ambition to discard the institutional tradition. But this was related only to people with a mild handicap. Those whose handicap was more severe were still restricted to being placed in one of the new residential institutions being built during a 20-year period which began in the mid-1950s.

In the 1967 Act living in one's own home, or in a group home, was still the only housing alternative outside the residential institution. It was not until the 1985 Act, with the establishment of a group home with extensive support, that people with a more severe handicap received the right to housing outside the institution. For the first time all people with intellectual handicap had the right to housing and a life outside the institution (Ericsson, 1986a).

The boarding house was the earliest form of housing with support outside the institution. Housing was provided in the home of a family, the parents providing the support for the person. During the 1960s this type of housing was extended. The group home came to comprise several apartments in one or more apartment blocks, support being provided by employed staff instead of the couple in a family (Palmér, 1974).

The person with handicap usually lived on their own in a small apartment, if it was larger it could be shared with a roommate. Normally, however, there was only a limited amount of staff support which meant that the person was expected to cope on their own. Because of the high demand placed on being able to cope, it was people with a mild handicap who lived in this type of housing.

The idea of a cluster of group homes, where several group homes could be established in a geographical area to form an administrative unit, was formulated in the early 1970s. A common staff group was responsible for the provision of support and service to the people living there (Stockholms läns landsting, 1977). The new element introduced was that staff support could be varied between the different group homes. Whereas people in one had staff support only in the mornings and evenings, another could have access to staff round-the-clock. With the establishment of this type of housing it became possible to provide support even for people with extensive needs, people who previously had been referred to institutional care.

This type of cluster of group homes included not only apartments but also detached housing. In this way suitable housing could be more easily found (Ericsson *et al.*, 1980). For example, houses away from the demands of the immediate neighbourhood made it possible to provide for those who wanted, or needed, some distance between themselves and their neighbours.

Different traditions have developed concerning the use of detached housing. In one type the private part is limited to the bedroom, while the bathroom, kitchen and sitting-room are shared. In another, the kitchen and a sitting-room are shared and each person has a small apartment with kitchen, sitting-room, bedroom and bathroom. There are usually 4-6 such apartments in this type of house (Socialstyrelsen, 1987).

There are now several types of housing available outside the residential institution. They vary in several ways, as regards the style of housing, location, proximity to neighbours, size of the private area and extent of staff support provided. The opportunity for personally planned housing has increased considerably, this being a basic requirement if alternatives to the traditional institution are to be realized (Ericsson, 1991). This pattern of housing is a consequence of developments which have taken place beginning with the first boarding houses of the 1940s. These have not only been influenced by changes within the services but also by external societal factors (Ericsson and Ericsson, 1988).

TWO WAYS OF LOOKING AT HOUSING

HOUSING ALTERNATIVES AFTER INSTITUTIONAL CLOSURE

When closing institutions questions arise concerning the location, the type of housing needed, and the extent of staff support. In an analysis of this Ericsson and Ericsson (1980) found critical differences concerning what was regarded as good housing for people with intellectual handicap. Three aspects were shown to differentiate between two views on housing. The first, 'should housing outside the institution be made available for all, or only for certain people?' was motivated by the doubt that existed as to whether all, or only those with a mild intellectual handicap, could live outside the institution after it had been closed. By tradition, and even in legislation in the 1954 Act, only the 'educable' had previously been given access to this type of housing, while the 'ineducable' had been referred to institutions. When institutional closure became a reality, and all were to move, the idea that life outside the institution was a privilege available only to those with a mild handicap, was clearly questioned.

The second question, 'should housing be anonymously, or personally planned?' was motivated by the tradition that residential facilities had been always anonymous. It should be possible for anyone to move to a placement in a residential institution. The third question, 'has the person the right to live permanently in their home?' grew out of the anxiety felt by relatives and staff, as to whether the person, after having moved from the institution, would have to move again. It was customary that people living in institutions would be moved between wards and even institutions, resulting in a life with many breaks from familiar surroundings.

As a consequence of the various answers to these questions one can find two ways of looking at housing. As housing alternatives developed, one model which emerged focused on training. This view expressed the idea of housing as a place with an educational content, with the purpose of having a developmental effect on the person. It provided an opportunity for training, something not previously available in the institution. Labels were used such as 'hygiene training', 'food training' and 'activities of daily living training', when describing the person's need to cope with personal hygiene in order to be clean, eating meals in order not to be hungry and participation in the care of the home because one lives there.

This view also expressed the idea that housing was for those only with enough competence to move from the institution. A life outside the institution was not therefore intended for all. Moving was regarded as a step in a 'career' between different units, with varying degrees of support on a ward or in the community, intended for those who were able to move on. It was therefore logical that this type of housing was anonymously planned, as different people should be able to avail themselves of the same housing. Neither was it self-evident that one had the right to stay on in the house in which one, for the time being, was resident.

A contrasting view was illustrated by the idea that a house should be the place where the person has their home. Life there should be similar to that led by a non-handicapped person. People acquire houses and create homes, not only by furnishing and equipping them according to individual wishes, but also by developing social relations and emotional security. It was through personally planned housing that these requirements could be met.

These two ways of looking at housing express different perspectives concerning both people with intellectual handicap and the services they receive (Kebbon, 1979). These two views can be termed the 'competence perspective' and the 'citizen perspective'. A similar discussion is found with Mercer's (1973) ideas on the clinical and the social perspective and Wolfensberger's (1969) way of looking at the social roles society gives this group of handicapped people and the different way services are developed (Ericsson and Ericsson, 1989).

THE COMPETENCE PERSPECTIVE

What here is called the competence perspective has its origins in the social roles of 'pupil' and 'patient'. They are associated with institutional patterns of service, education and care being the two main forms provided. Depending on whether a person was seen as 'educable' or 'ineducable', they were referred to different institutions. The 'educable' left for the school institution, were designated the role of 'pupil' and provided with education, The 'ineducable' were admitted to asylums, later residential institutions, where a more medically-orientated form of care was dominant, especially after the 1954 Act. There the social role of 'patient' was dominant.

Even if these two roles are very different, their common feature is that both focus on the person's lack of competence. A 'pupil' lacks knowledge and must therefore be educated and a 'patient' lacks basic functions which could be developed through care practices. The common feature of these social roles was that different measures were taken to increase competence.

These measures were organized by specialized bodies, in specialized premises and environments (such as special schools, residential institutions or specialized housing, group homes or day activity centres). The greater part of their task was aimed at increasing people's independence and preparing them for participation in community life. In this case participation in the life of the community only becomes possible when the person is considered to have achieved the level of competence required to meet the demands of society.

THE CITIZEN PERSPECTIVE

The citizen perspective is based on the social role of 'citizen' as expressed in the development of the normalization principle of 1946. The aspect being focused on here is that the person with intellectual handicap is first of all a citizen, like all others born into this society. Thus the rights and obligations which apply for others are equally applicable. However, because of their disability, the person with intellectual handicap also needs support and service from others in order to participate in the life of society.

The question of the person's influence over their own life is, in this perspective, an important issue. So is their need for support if they are to exercise that influence. When it comes to achieving a good life, it is the person's own idea of what is considered a good life which must be the basis for the service provided. Support and services need to be provided on individual terms if they are to contribute to the realization of the kind of life the person wishes to live. If the person's own wishes are the starting point, the premises and environments of the service organizations are not likely to be where they choose to live. Instead it is often the ordinary environments and social situations of society which are sought. The task of providing support and service must, therefore, out of necessity, take place in the ordinary community. The task becomes one of making such environments accessible and adjusting them to the needs of the person with intellectual handicap: of creating personal living environments.

But given this perspective what place is there for a concern about enhancing competence? Since the person does have a disability this remains an important goal: the question which arises is how is this to be achieved and, in particular, how are the individual's views to be respected?

Within the framework of the normalization process described earlier, a change also occurs concerning the perception by society of people with intellectual handicap. The competence perspective and the citizen perspective as presented here, express the nature of this change.

HOUSING AND A HOME FROM THE CITIZEN PERSPECTIVE

There is already extensive experience of developing housing for people with intellectual handicap based on the competence perspective, this having been the prevailing view in services with an institutional tradition. It is more difficult to find examples of the use of the citizen perspective. In the remaining part of this chapter some of the key areas are identified to which attention must be given in the process of establishing housing, a home and a life in the community (Ericsson, 1989).

What is needed is housing for people with various kinds of handicaps. Some have grown up within the family, others in institutions, some have a mild handicap while others are more severely disabled. As the right to housing outside the institution applies to everyone, the challenge is to develop housing and a home for all. Those with a severe handicap in particular, are people with unique needs, therefore, unique ways of providing support and service must be found if their needs are to be met. A wide variety of housing is therefore necessary if the multi-faceted needs are to be met. That is why there is a need for a model to create individually-tailored housing. If the task is to achieve personal housing, then it must start with the needs of the person, or possibly the group, who are to live there. One must know, therefore, at an early stage who is going to live there.

When looking for a house the same conditions apply for a person with intellectual handicap as for a non-handicapped person. It is a sensitive task which requires a number of important decisions and needs support from people who can contribute towards accomplishing the task, i.e. the family, bank contacts and housing agencies are some of those who have a role to play.

For a person with intellectual handicap there is also the difficulty of expressing oneself and asserting one's interest. As many are unable to express their opinions in these matters an advocate is necessary who can capture, describe and express the needs of the person. Even if the person can express their own views they may need someone who can be of moral support in discussions about their housing requirements.

Acquiring a house is only part of the larger task of settling in a community, establishing social relationships and creating a life. It is also a question of what the individual wants to do during the day, in the evenings and at weekends, and where they want to live, and with whom.

An understanding of what sort of life the person wishes to live cannot of course be achieved at a first meeting, but will be the subject of many discussions. The suggestions which will result from these discussions will probably not coincide with the wishes originally expressed. These meetings will often be characterized as negotiations where realistic and short- term decisions must be reached so that support and service can be made available.

Collectively, those concerned must be able to find solutions while at the same time recognizing existing limitations for the satisfaction of personal needs and wishes. Throughout, one must also be able to continue long-term discussions about the life the person wishes to live.

A matter about which agreement must be reached is the place where the person is to live. Is it in a district where many forms of service are available already or do they wish to live in their original community, for example, where parents and family now live?

When the district has been decided, there is a need to decide upon the neighbourhood. Does the person wish to live in an existing housing area, on the outskirts of a residential area at a comfortable distance from neighbours, or in the countryside? The type of housing existing in the district will, in the end, determine how the person will live. Only if that housing does not meet the requirements of the residents should special housing be built.

At present the special services that arrange housing for people with handicaps are also the owners of the property. This is natural as residential services were previously provided in the form of residential institutions. It was almost unthinkable that this housing could and would eventually be owner-occupied. With increasing awareness that ordinary housing in the community, with suitable adjustment, can be used for people with intellectual handicap requirements for the development of housing have also changed. A family can now give their son or daughter support to create housing and a home, in the same way they would for a son or daughter without handicap.

A critical factor which determines whether a person can live under these conditions is whether they have access to adequate personal support. If they receive support from other people then they can live under such conditions, if not, then their possibilities of experiencing this type of life are limited. Those with the task of providing support are usually specially employed staff and questions arise concerning their number, training, working methods and other formal matters such as terms of employment.

But there are also other people. When support and service is provided outside the institution others who are familiar with the community also have experience and knowledge which can contribute towards a more fulfilled life. The family and relatives of service users have a contribution to make, as do advocates and others who are involved in enabling them to establish participation in the life of the community. It is also important to develop a secure and stable relationship with neighbours, without the individuals concerned having to feel questioned or threatened. It is also possible to create a support group to the group home, whose function is to ensure good relations, in the house and in the contact of the group with the community.

A house can be developed into a home, where the person can create a life for themselves. The home can become the place where they live their private life, concerned with their own well-being, not least their most private activities which go on behind a locked door. It is in their own home that it is possible to express their most personal views about what has happened during the day, without being questioned. This is the place where they can feel free and secure. It is also here that they look after their own needs, for example their appearance and their clothing, and undertake household jobs in the private as well as shared areas. Recreation and hobbies, friends and relaxation are also part of home life. Housing is also the platform from which they establish participation in community life, preparing to make purchases, caring for their health and well-being, taking part in culture and recreation as well as social relations and community involvement.

A TWO-DIMENSIONAL DEVELOPMENT OF SERVICES

As a number of other contributors have noted (Chapters 4 and 5), the dramatic changes taking place in the type of services do not necessarily bring about a changed perception of people with intellectual handicap, their relation to society or to the services provided (Ericsson and Ericsson, 1989). The development can be simply illustrated by a two-dimensional matrix (Figure 6.1).

The starting point for the normalization process can be seen in square A. The care provided in the residential institution was associated with the competence perspective, that is the roles of 'pupil' and 'patient'. The series of residential institutions which were established from the mid-1950s had, for example, a pronounced medical character, having been built as modified versions of hospitals. The role of 'patient' was therefore natural in these places.

A development away from this position could lead in three directions.

	Competence Perspective	Citizen Perspective
Institutional Support	A	B
Community Support	C	D

Figure 6.1 Two perspectives on residential services.

From square A to square B would lead to an entirely different type of institution whose content was based on the citizen perspective. However, it has never been suggested that the residential institutions or the special services be changed in this direction, even if it would have been possible. Instead the decision has been made to close institutions and replace them with a community system of services.

With the normalization principle of 1946 as one starting point and the role of citizen as a basis for community services as the other, the process of change within the services should give rise to a shift from institutional to community services on the one hand, and from the competence perspective to that of the citizen perspective on the other. In the matrix this would be indicated by a shift from A towards D.

An analysis of the two perspectives on housing has shown, however, the occurrence of other alternatives. If the task has only been to change the form of the services, without regard to the content, the result would be a shift from A towards C, community services being run from the competence perspective.

In the everyday task of running services these are important questions which often give rise to uncertainty and disputes. This is especially noticeable in discussions on working methods, questions of staff qualifications or when different viewpoints are expressed in staff groups. There are few who defend the existence of large institutions so the conflict between institutional and community services is uncommon. Instead there is a collision between the different perspectives from which people with intellectual handicap are viewed within community services.

CONCLUSION

The implications of the citizen perspective remain to be fully explored. It is not clear that this perspective is yet considered desirable by public services organizations. Within a service with a long tradition, characterized by institutional patterns with a pronounced hierarchical structure, many challenges to these new ideas arise. Basically it is a question of how one perceives people with intellectual handicap, their families and relatives, who share in the task of forming services for those with intellectual handicap.

If one does intend to run services from the citizen perspective the question also arises about how changes should take place. In an organization focused on economic and administrative aspects of providing services there may be limited experience of how to go about changing views. There are those who even doubt that this is possible. Karan *et al.*, (1992) consider that the development of 'supported living' – their expression for a system of providing housing characterized by the citizen perspective – implies nothing less than a revolution for traditional service providers. To develop a citizen perspective requires a humble attitude towards those to whom support is being offered, as well as a critical approach towards the history of the service organization and present-day practices. As fewer of those requesting support and service in the form of housing come from institutions, and an increasing number have previously lived in their parental homes, more demands are being made that the housing provided be developed from the citizen perspective.

The 1946 principle of normalization gives the citizen perspective another function. The socio-political idea which normalization represents has sometimes been found to be difficult to understand and has given rise to extensive debate. During the process of change it has often been applied in a mechanical and administrative manner. The mere existence of these two perspectives can be seen as an expression of the lack of clarity concerning the intentions and content of the normalization process. A manifestation of the citizen perspective could be a contribution towards the clarification of the principle of normalization. The consequences of the citizen perspective, as suggested here, have bearing not only on the content of existing housing but even give rise to alternative ideas as to how more appropriate housing could be developed.

The housing most commonly produced in Sweden today consists of separate apartments with adjoining common facilities, usually built as detached housing but sometimes developed within an apartment block. Their construction is derived from the aspiration to provide as much private space as possible, but within the framework of a specially designed house or part of an apartment block. It is appreciated by many and has provided new opportunities for people to acquire housing and a home. But looking at this situation from the citizen perspective, this continues to be anonymously planned housing, designed according to directives decided by national bodies and built throughout the country. Only occasionally does the building style reflect the character of the neighbour-hood. The person who is going to live there seldom has any influence over the design of the housing which can therefore be seen as a standard-ized apartment in a public service unit.

It is surprising that this type of housing is being developed at a time when so many are moving from the residential institution: people with the most complex disabilities and the most unique personal needs. When the need for personally planned housing is greatest, housing should be designed to meet a diversity of individual needs, however, only one type of standard housing intended for all is being offered. The debate about the meaning of personally planned housing and having a home of one's own, must therefore continue. Experience must also be gained in order to throw light on what demands must be made if this goal is to be realized. The question of the availability of personally planned housing for the intellectually disabled and the aquisition of owner-occupied homes is still waiting for an answer.

Supported living policies and programmes in the USA 7

Mary Ann Allard

In the early 1980s, community residential services for people with mental retardation or developmental disabilities in the United States began to change from an often rigid, unresponsive, programme or facility approach in residential services to an individualized and supportive approach to community living. This chapter addresses an innovative approach that emanated from these concerns, usually described as 'supported living'. The chapter is presented in four parts:

1. The major forces that have shaped supported living in the United States today.
2. A definition of supported living and how it differs from traditional residential service programmes together with examples of supported living programmes in the United States.
3. Selected findings from existing studies of supported living.
4. Questions/issues that should be addressed in a future research agenda concerning this approach to community life.

FORCES THAT HAVE SHAPED SUPPORTED LIVING POLICIES AND PROGRAMMES

Although individuals lived in the community with various types and amounts of support before the 1980s, the term 'supported living' did not exist in the lexicon of community residential services until the mid-1980s. In their analysis of trends in community residential services, Lakin *et al.* (1988) added an important residential category – 'supported independent living' – to their well-known classification of community-based residential programmes and noted that this category had not been subject to national research or data collection efforts.

The next section considers six forces which have shaped supported living policies and programmes:

- the critique of excessive individualization;
- shifting government from provision to enabling;
- reassessment of what it means to be in the community;
- criticism of the developmental continuum;
- a crisis in resourcing;
- changing definitions of mental retardation.

THE CRITIQUE OF EXCESSIVE INDIVIDUALIZATION

During the 1980s, dissatisfaction with the emerging form and content of community services coincided with wider political re-evaluation of the role of government, from both ends of the political spectrum. Several critics of American mental retardation/developmental disabilities policy have noted the need for a similar approach used by critics of the broader social policy framework that focuses on the need for a 'communitarian' alternative (Bellah *et al.*, 1985). Bellah *et al.* suggest that the individualistic traditions in American society have made it difficult to develop a commitment to others, and has led to isolation from our families, community institutions, and political parties, among others (as cited in Turnbull, 1991). From the disability/mental retardation perspective, Turnbull (1991, p.24) stresses that we should focus less on liberty and autonomy of individuals and more on community and 'the common good of all of us' and Ferguson *et al.* (1990, p.15) argue that 'excessive individualism in disability policies and services are closely related to the role of client and the dependency status often encouraged by that role'.

Bellah *et al.* (1991, p.26, cited in Turnbull, 1991) point out that community entities such as churches and synagogues, schools, voluntary organizations, are mediating structures and that 'only greater citizen participation in the large structure of the economy and the state will help us surmount the deepening problems of contemporary social life'. McKnight (1987, p. 56) suggests that community – 'the social place used by family, friends, neighbours, neighbourhood groups and associations, ethnic associations, temples, churches, local union, local government ... and [which can] also be described as informal, unmanaged and associational – has been ignored because institutional leaders do not believe in the capacities of communities and since most are part of hierarchical systems, all authority, resources, and dollars flow away from communities to service systems.

The individualistic tradition also fosters self-centredness that gets in the way of focusing on care and responsibility for others (Turnbull, 1991). Conversely, community living works best when individuals stop thinking of themselves as the centre of the universe: Kendrick (1989, p.25) suggests that there is a need for personal sacrifice on behalf of others and that change must occur not only in the external world but also within ourselves. In other words, simply changing the rules by which we relate to community and individuals may not be enough – these changes must be internalized to make them real and authentic.

SHIFTING GOVERNMENT FROM PROVISION TO ENABLING

Another trend that parallels the criticism of the American social and legal structure can be traced to the business literature. Much of this discussion has revolved around how to define and create 'quality'. In brief, these business ideas have been adapted by political analysts and applied to government bureaucracy. As noted by Osborne (1992), in order to be more responsive to consumer needs, governments must be 'flexible, adaptable, ... decentralised and innovative' instead of hierarchical and centralized. Governments can become more entrepreneurial, that is, more consumer oriented by acting as catalysts, brokers and 'steering' society rather than 'rowing'. These types of governments must also be focused on outcomes that tell the consumer what he or she is getting for the social and economic investments made in various programmes. Are persons with mental retardation living in publicly-funded community residences satisfied with the quality of their lives?

The extent to which compliance with government regulations actually leads to quality in residential life has been the subject of a symposium sponsored by the American Association on Mental Retardation (AAMR) (Mental Retardation Vol. 30, June 1992), in which the general consensus was that regulation and oversight in residential life for persons with mental retardation has not led to quality. Although much of this discussion was focused on the most heavily regulated federal/state residential programme in the United States, the Medicaid funded Intermediate Care Facility for the Mentally Retarded (ICF/MR) programme, the thrust of this ongoing debate is directly relevant to innovative approaches such as supported living. Firstly, 'regulatory intervention is competing with the aspirations and contemporary values embodied in the new support paradigm' (Holburn, 1992, p.130). Secondly, the adherence to a professionally driven individual service plan without including some type of 'person-centred planning' perpetuates the notion that professionals must 'cure or fix' people with disabilities before they are ready to live the kind of life they want to live (Shea, 1992, p.147). And thirdly, the organizational implications of a shift to a third phase, i.e., the supports stage, stresses a structure that is not characterized by professional bureaucracies governed by regulations, centralization and hierarchy but rather an 'organic' control model that is 'designed around values, informal norms of behaviours and interpersonal communication rather than formal rules and documentation' (Gardner, 1992, p.75).

Some of the structural changes in community residential services that are emerging out of the forces identified above include:

- using a different approach to planning for the individual with mental retardation – one that includes attention to lifestyles and/or 'futures' issues, that is, a focus on individual 'gifts' and capacity instead of deficits and remediation of those deficits;
- changing the way in which human service organisations are structured to respond to individuals and to create flexible and tailored supports to meet their lifestyle choices;
- empowering and valuing not only persons with disabilities but also staff that will be part of this new social order (Smull, 1993).

REASSESSING WHAT IT MEANS TO BE IN THE COMMUNITY

Some of the concerns reported in the literature regarding community living for persons with disabilities, especially for those persons who were previously institutionalized, include their lack of social integration, isolation and loneliness despite their physical presence in the community (Bercovici, 1983). Further, it has been reported that persons with mental retardation usually lacked community connections (Taylor et al., 1987) friendships, other than with paid staff, (Specht and Nagy, 1986; Romer and Heller, 1983) and opportunities to exercise choices or make decisions about all aspects of their daily lives (Halpern et al., 1986). Alternative approaches to just being in the community have included a shift from programme planning to more creative individualized planning and rethinking what quality of life really means and how to enable persons with mental retardation to achieve a desired lifestyle. O'Brien (1987) describes five accomplishments or outcomes that constitute a quality life: community presence, choice, competence, respect and community participation. These five components have been used increasingly at the local level to develop individual lifestyle planning and at the state level to help guide mental retardation services systems.

CRITICISM OF THE DEVELOPMENTAL CONTINUUM

Since the early 1960s, the community residential services system in the

United States has been governed by a concept known as the 'continuum of care' (President's Panel on Mental Retardation, 1962). Although the original conceptualization of the continuum envisaged individuals drawing from an array of services depending on their needs, the theory was interpreted by residential planners like a 'stepladder; each rung of the ladder represents a living arrangement whose purpose is to teach the client the skills needed to ascend to the next step' (Johnson, 1985). In short, it was assumed that individuals with mental retardation must possess certain prerequisite skills (e.g. cooking, shopping) before 'progressing' to the next least restrictive environment and with that earning the right to basic human goals, such as living in one's own home or having control over daily decisions.

The residential continuum was interpreted as meaning that people must 'get ready' to move to less restrictive living arrangements and must be able to meet the entrance and exit criteria tied to specialized programmes. In general, persons with severe disabilities never moved to less restrictive settings, while others had to move continually in order to reach more desirable goals, such as greater freedom and responsibility (Taylor, 1988; Klein, 1992).

Critics of this approach have designed services so that, although individuals with mental retardation do draw from an array of services (such as financial, vocational, respite, mobility, community, medical care and others), services begin with the individual and their needs, personal preferences and choices. In addition, unlike the traditional residential continuum, services and supports are brought to the individual in his or her own home (or other community place), are flexible, and can be modified to reflect changes in level of intensity of need so that the staff supports move instead of the individual (Dufresne, 1992; Shearer, 1986).

CRISIS IN RESOURCING

Fuelling the critique of the existing residential services system are several hard realities. Firstly, there simply is not enough capacity in the existing residential system (staff, funding and programme alternatives) to meet the needs of all people with mental retardation/developmental disabilities (Smull, 1989). Amado and Heal (1990) note that the availability of residential beds has decreased by nearly 13% over the last decade. Secondly, it is clear that purchasing programmes (entire services) on behalf of individuals who need only targeted services or supports, such as transportation or meals, was inefficient and leading to serious fiscal inequities in service delivery. In the United States, the majority of federal/state funds in mental retardation or developmental disabilities support a relatively small number of individuals (Braddock *et al.*, 1990). As Smull (1989) puts it: 'There's a crisis and there is no way existing resources can meet al. l of the expectations'.

CHANGING DEFINITION OF MENTAL RETARDATION

The American Association on Mental Retardation, the largest professional organization representing various disciplines in mental retardation in the United States, recently adopted a new definition of mental retardation that focuses on the intensity of supports needed rather than an IQ-derived level of retardation. Instead of using existing subcategories of mild, moderate, severe and profound, the new definition suggests that an individual's support needs may range from intermittent to extensive and may be lifelong (AAMR, 1992).

A DEFINITION OF SUPPORTED LIVING

In the United States, the mental retardation services system has gone through two distinct historical phases: the first phase focused on institutionalization and segregation and the second stage on deinstitutionalization and community services. Precipitated by the 'community crisis' alluded to above, the next, and some think the final stage, in the development of residential services has been described as one of community membership and functional supports (Smull and Bellamy, 1991; Bradley and Knoll, 1991; Taylor *et al.*, 1987). Instead of creating specially designed residences or making individuals adapt to their environments, the intent is to move supports to where people live and to adapt their environment and supports to them. The concept of functional supports is an alternative to forcing individuals to fit into available programme 'slots' and to consider creating a network of formal and informal supports that a person needs to live in his or her community (Smith, 1991; Bradley and Knoll, 1991).

Supported living is a relatively new and evolving concept. As noted by Klein (1991, p.1), it is a philosophy and approach; it is 'not a model, the answer or some new magic. It is, however, a way of viewing people and assisting them in ways that enable them to receive supports they need to live in a home they want'. Although there continues to be some debate, supported living can be defined as enabling people, regardless of their disabilities, to live in the community where they want, with whom they want, for as long as they want, and with whatever supports they need to do that (Shearer, 1986; Ferguson *et al.*, 1990; Karan and Granfield, 1990).

From this definition follow a number of important principles or values:

- developing an individually-based plan, not facility or programme-based planning;
- creating flexible supports and services;
- enabling and supporting choices that individuals make;
- enabling individuals to control their own homes;
- assisting and developing connections to the community;
- separating housing from support and services;
- developing funding that is individually- not programme-based;
- using both informal and formal supports that blend together creative, naturalistic and less bureaucratic responses to individual needs;
- including all persons with mental retardation/developmental disabilities.

Some analysts would suggest that supported living is primarily focused on individual choice and control/ownership of the home where they live (Karan *et al.*, 1992). Others would include a list of principles and values, such as the one highlighted above, and would add a principle that addresses the fundamental restructuring of formal residential agencies to become a 'support provider' (O'Brien and Lyle O'Brien, 1991; Knoll, 1992). In a recent exploration of supported living in five states, Burwell *et al.* (1993) found a wide range of interpretations of supported living, but among the key components 'having choices' was the first and foremost principle.

As Taylor (1991) notes in a review of certain individualized community living arrangements in Wisconsin:

> The concept is deceptively simple – find a home, whether a house, apartment or other dwelling, and build in the staff supports necessary for the person to live successfully in the community. Inherent in the concept is flexibility. Some people may need only part-time supports or merely someone to drop by to make sure they are okay. Others with severe disabilities and challenging needs may require full-time staff support. There isn't anything in the concept that precludes small groups of people from living together ... this, however, should be because they choose to live together and are compatible.
>
> (Taylor, 1991, p.108)

A SNAPSHOT OF SUPPORTED LIVING PROGRAMMES IN THE USA

According to some individuals who have been closely involved either in assisting or monitoring the implementation of supported living, no one state has redesigned its entire community residential system to focus on supportive living (Klein, 1991; Smith, 1990). Although there is no formal estimate of the number of individuals participating in supported living programmes across the United States, in 1988, 17 000 individuals were living in semi-independent or supported living (Wright *et al.*, 1991). The inclusion of semi-independent programmes is problematic since in many residential conceptualizations this represents the last rung on the continuum ladder before complete independence and the programme criteria may not reflect the values/principles associated with supported living. Similarly, this estimate may include supported living programmes that do not meet the basic principles noted earlier.

In 1991, Smith highlighted eight states that served the following number of persons with mental retardation/developmental disabilities in distinct supported living programmes:

- Illinois: Community Integrated Living Arrangements – 1000 (including persons with mental illness);
- Colorado: Personal Care Alternatives – 700;
- Washington: Tenant Support – 1000;
- Minnesota: Supported Living Arrangement – 1400;
- North Dakota: Individualized Supported Living Arrangement – 600;
- Florida: Supported Living Program (formerly the Supported Independent Living Program) – 500 individuals but soon to expand significantly with a recently approved federal waiver for community-based services);
- Ohio-Supported Living – 1500;
- Wisconsin: Community Integration Program – of the 2000 people with disabilities receiving services in 1992, approximately 35% (700) are in supported living programmes. Another significant resource for supported living is the 'Community Aide' programme, a 'block grant' of state and other dollars – approximately 1800 are in supported living.

These estimates total approximately 9200 people. In addition, many other states, including Georgia, Maryland, New Hampshire, Nevada, Oklahoma, Virginia, Oregon and Michigan, have recently initiated supported living programmes. As such, the true number of supported living participants is likely to be higher.

To date, supported living programmes in the United States have been financed through two major sources: state general revenues and the federal/state Medicaid Home and Community Based (HCB) waiver programme. In 1990, the United States Congress passed an amendment to the federal Medicaid law allowing states to compete for a new Medicaid option called Community Supported Living Arrangements (CSLA).

Although this was a limited and targeted amount of federal dollars available (approximately $100 million in total is available for five years in eight states), it represented the first time that the federal government became a player in the expansion of supportive living. Prior to the enactment of CSLA, many states were using the HCB waiver to serve persons with mental retardation/developmental disabilities, especially those with more severe disabilities, in various supported living arrangements. Since 27 states applied for one of the eight CSLA grants available, it is evident that there is significant interest in either expanding or developing greater individualized and supported living options for persons with mental retardation.

Smith (1990) divided the type of financing for supported living into those resources targeted to 'housing and other living expenses' and those targeted to 'support services'. The former is primarily funded through various social insurance entitlements and private and public housing subsidies, while the latter is financed through the HCB waiver, other Medicaid 'optional' services such as personal care attendants, and state revenues (the federal/state Medicaid programme prohibits payment for room and board). Since one of the principles and objectives of providing supports to individuals living in the community is to remove the deleterious effects of payment based on a programme or facility, the mechanisms used to finance supported living reflect this approach.

In order to illustrate some of the ways in which states have implemented the principles of supported living, several descriptive examples are provided below (descriptions after Smith (1990) and Taylor *et al.* (1991)).

Colorado's Personal Care Alternatives (PCA) programme was stimulated by one agency's conversion from a traditional continuum to residential supports in homes controlled by the individual. The PCA programme allows community agencies to use both Medicaid dollars and the individual's own resources to provide support in non-group home settings in which no more than two persons with developmental disabilities live. Peer companion, supported apartments and host homes are used as supported living options. Anyone can be a candidate for the PCA placement, and a recent evaluation demonstrated that persons served in the supported living option were not significantly different from people served in more conventional residences.

Wisconsin's Options in Community Living – perhaps the oldest example of a residential programme to offer only individualized support services – has influenced a state-wide community integration programme. Options began in 1974 as a component of a larger agency and was incorporated as an independent agency in 1981. It is committed to the ideal that any person, no matter what the nature of his or her disability, can live in a supported living environment. Both Washington and Minnesota have a two-tier supportive living programme: one level that focuses on people that need less than 24-hour supervision and can manage somewhat independently and another level for those with more intensive supports or who need continuous daily assistance.

All of these states and Florida's Supported Living (FSL) programme have the individual with a disability play a central role in defining his or her personal goals. FSL includes a personal futures plan that is drafted collaboratively with a case manager, friends, family members and a supportive living 'coach'. Florida, Colorado and Wisconsin are developing quality assurance programmes that focus on the individual's quality of life. For example, FSL has designed a handbook for monitoring quality of life that is targeted at individuals and their designated volunteers. Several other states (e.g. Maryland) have used a similar strategy to indicate quality of life outcomes.

Supported living programmes usually involve innovative funding strategies. North Dakota's Individualised Supported Living Arrangements Program serves individuals in apartments or homes of their own choice and develops funding rates that are unique to the individual. Payments for the services detailed in each individual service plan are linked to a contract and an individualized daily rate for habilitation or personal care (the former entails a focus on training whereas the latter is more or less supports or services to maintain and enhance an individual's ability to live a quality of life). There is no overall payment cap or ceiling on programme rates, though there are limits on provider agency administrative costs. If savings are achieved, the providers benefit economically. Further, North Dakota adjusts more than 500 rates twice a year – a by-product of reviewing individual service plans every six months. Daily rates range from $10–$286.

In Colorado, rates vary depending on the use of live-in assistants or roommates. In 1990, the average payment for a PCA placement averaged $58.93/day (this includes both the services portion and the individual's paid room and board charges and local matching funds). At the high end, average payments totalled $91.10/day with $35.75/day at the low end. Wisconsin and Illinois essentially use a capitation method whereby community agencies/county governments, respectively, are given a uniform or per capita dollar amount for a range of services to all supported living participants served by an agency/county. Agencies/counties can then allocate the funds on an individual basis by constructing customized service packages from a menu of services.

These projects also emphasize the development of connections with the community and use both informal and formal supports. North Dakota puts strong emphasis on using natural, or unpaid, supports available in the community as does Wisconsin's community integration programme, including friends, neighbours, and family members and other local sources of support. For example, in Florida's supported living programme, some agencies have used generic, or non-specialized funding sources, such as adult education, to hire 'community living instructors'. These individuals not only support individuals both in their home and during the day, but they facilitate necessary community connections. For example, community living instructors serve as guides or, as some authors describe, bridge-builders to community establishments such as the local grocery store and the bank. In many instances, these community entities become part of the informal support network for the individual, e.g. personnel in one bank in Florida provide the money management assistance for an individual who cannot perform those tasks independently.

For the most part, states have established supportive living initiatives without requiring specific legislation. A few states such as Maryland and Illinois have passed legislation specifying the philosophy, values and intent of supportive living. Maryland's statute affirms that all persons including those with severe disabilities are eligible for community supported living services. Although few states have enacted specific mandates establishing a supported living approach, many states have recently revised or adopted new mission statements guiding all mental retardation/developmental disabilities policies at the state level. The values stated usually highlight many of the components of supported living and direct quality assurance activities to reflect personal outcomes, such as honouring individual choices and empowering individuals in their daily lives (Connecticut Department of Mental Retardation, 1987). The extent to which states are living up to these values has not been evaluated.

SELECTED FINDINGS FROM A FIVE-STATE STUDY

Burwell *et al.* (1993) carried out a study of supported living in five states for the United States Department of Health and Human Services, Assistant Secretary for Planning and Evaluation (ASPE). The objectives of this policy study were to analyse supported living in a sample of states and to develop some recommendations regarding future federal policy on supported living. At the time of the study, the eight CSLA states were only just beginning to develop their programmes and information on their implementation was therefore largely speculative.

CONTEXT FOR SUPPORTED LIVING

The authors found that across the five states there were certain prerequisites to the development and acceptance of supported living. Firstly, there was a philosophical commitment to the underlying components of supported living. Most of these states had adopted the fundamental principles of supported living and encouraged their implementation, reflected in various ways: in agency policies, procedures, regulations and manuals; sponsoring conferences, workshops and symposia; and giving local agencies flexibility in meeting traditional accountability measures such as in licensing, quality assurance standards and payment of services. In several states, including Maryland and Florida, there was extensive collaboration among government, university and/or advocacy organizations regarding the implementation of supported living.

Secondly, the growth of supported employment influenced where people lived. It was clear to many key informants that the progress being made in supported employment would ultimately influence how and where people with disabilities lived in the community. As one state official noted, people with mental retardation were being supported during the day in integrated work settings but going back to the group home at night and forced to live by rules that were not of their choice (e.g. curfews, bathing schedules, no key to the front door).

Thirdly, State Developmental Disabilities Councils played key roles in the expansion of supported living. In four states, these federally funded state entities provided instrumental support to the concept of supported living. For example, 'systems change' or start-up grants were made to local agencies interested either in developing entirely new supported living programmes or in converting their traditional residential programmes to a supports approach (Illinois, Maryland). In Florida, the Developmental Disability Council funded a key staff person in state government to develop and implement a supported living model. These entities also provided training and technical assistance to local organizations developing supported living initiatives.

Fourthly, legislation on supported living was enacted. Although this observation was not found in all of the states, both Maryland and Ohio had separate mandates regarding supported living. In Maryland, the statute specified that supported living would be available to anyone, including persons with severe cognitive impairments and in Ohio, a separate funding appropriation was included for supported living. Key informants in several states indicated that a legislative base on supported living ensured a broader representation of programme participants and stability for the programme.

It was evident that some of the supported living programmes in the study were implementing the values of supported living with a greater commitment than others. Best practice was observed in three particular areas; individualization, choice and development.

The researchers found that staff in the best supported living programmes talked about individuals and told stories; they did not present organizational charts or assessment forms. The person with mental retardation was not seen as a client or resident but as a member of his or her community, someone they have responsibility to, not for (Smull, 1993). Staff in these programmes spend a long time getting to know the individuals whose lives they are helping to support; they listen to them carefully, either through their verbal or other means of expression. Staff with the Wisconsin Options in Community Living agency believe that it has taken them ten years to really get to know the individuals they support. Another support agency in rural Wisconsin noted that 'it took three years of meeting with consumers and families and listening to them to set up this programme'.

In many supported living programmes, some type of person-centred planning process (e.g. personal futures plan, essential lifestyle plan) was involved. As highlighted by many key informants, it is extremely useful for persons involved with supporting individuals with mental retardation/developmental disabilities to look at and think about this person in a different approach, that is, to see beyond skill deficits and deficiencies. According to Smull (1993), this process should include five elements:

- listening to the individuals or their representatives;
- identifying their preferences and core values;
- addressing the issues that the disability presents;
- developing a vision;
- mobilizing community resources to make that vision a reality.

Maryland, Florida and Wisconsin have encouraged supported living agencies either to adopt this type of planning process or a related version.

Good services honoured and encouraged individual choice and control over all aspects of daily living and integrated it into service design and plans. Individuals with mental retardation/developmental disabilities had meaningful choices about where they wanted to live, with whom and how they controlled their own housing. In these programmes, agencies did not own or lease the individual's home; in some cases, they did act as a guarantor on a lease or if the agency did own the home, they worked hard on transferring ownership to the individual(s) with mental retardation. Several agencies in the study states either rented residential property or their Board of Directors agreed, and sometimes were anxious, to 'get out of the real estate business'. For other agencies that were more heavily capitalized, providing home ownership to individuals with disabilities was a significant barrier.

Another barrier to individual control was money management. Key informants noted that this 'skill area' was particularly troublesome for many individuals with mental retardation, and in some cases, individuals could control their own housing but the service provider was still managing their money. Agencies did not like this conflict in roles and were investigating other ways in which support could be provided to help individuals with money management (e.g. some have either hired or asked bank personnel to perform some of these tasks).

Choices and options also extended to who should provide services to individuals with mental retardation/developmental disabilities. As others have stated, the ultimate sense of control for a client of the human services system, is to be able to 'hire and fire' those individuals who provide services to him or her. As part of Maryland's CSLA programme, individuals will be able to fire their service provider. In Ohio and Florida, individuals in supported living arrangements can fire their staff, but not usually the provider. In these cases, the service provider together with the individual will identify other staff or supports if the individual is not satisfied with the services.

The process of identifying and implementing informed choices for persons with mental retardation/developmental disabilities can be a complicated and risky endeavour. The supported living agencies that met this challenge stressed that they remain engaged with individuals when they made choices with adverse consequences. This process of engagement could span significant amounts of time and include consequences such as spending time in a homeless shelter or in jail. Key informants did not have answers that could be generalized to other individuals in risky choice-making situations since they noted that each individual is different.

Understanding how to provide supports to individuals with mental retardation/developmental disabilities is a slow process. Several key informants indicated that some local agencies cannot make this change and learn how to 'let people go'. Others noted that this approach may be best suited for non-traditional, creative organizations, and in some cases, that may mean building an entirely new organization devoted to supporting individuals in the community. At the same time, the principles of supported living can easily be lost in the translation from theory to practice. For example, in Illinois, the Community Integrated Living Arrangements (CILA) programme became a variation of the group home model with 24-hour staffing, structured schedules and limited privacy. One local agency in Florida described some of its programmes as 'pre-supported living'.

CHARACTERISTICS OF INDIVIDUALS IN SUPPORTED LIVING PROGRAMMES

Many of the individuals visited in the five states received intermittent supports/services. Supported living options were being used by a variety of individuals with disabilities especially:

- persons who were older and living in their own home after many years of institutionalization;
- persons with challenging behaviours and mental health problems who have been excluded from many continuum programmes and now had a place of their own with control over who was involved in their lives;
- persons with medical needs and/or severe cognitive impairments.

For those individuals who were unable to express or to make their choices known, either an advocate, close friend or family member assisted in those areas.

It was also evident that in some programmes, especially if persons with severe cognitive disabilities were involved, the supported living option looked and felt different with respect to the degree of choice and risk taking allowed, the opportunities for integration and the imposition of regulations and standards. One of these examples was found in Illinois where supported living agencies began to change as they accepted persons moving out of nursing homes who required 24-hour care. In other states, the ability to include persons with more severe disabilities was limited by financial resources; for example, Florida's supported living option was restricted to persons requiring less than 24 hours support, but recent changes in its Medicaid Home and Community-Based waiver will allow the state to include persons with more intensive needs. In general, however, most key informants felt that anyone could participate in supported living options if sufficient resources were available.

CHARACTERISTICS OF SUPPORTED LIVING ORGANIZATIONS AND THEIR STAFF

The study team identified three basic organizational approaches to supported living in the five states: the agency team model, the county operated model and the multi-team model.

Maryland, Florida and Wisconsin all had examples of the agency team model. In this model, a team of supported living workers are supervised by a programme director. The primary emphasis is for the support worker to develop a peer relationship with the person receiving the support. One support agency used a self-management team of five house counsellors to support not only the person in his/her home but also each other. The range of responsibilities of support workers was very broad, including applying for benefits for the individual and finding housing, dealing with landlords, introducing people to their neighbours, assisting with job searches, going shopping together and eating out. The job description of a supported living worker has been summarized as: 'Whatever needs to be done – do it'.

Many states in the United States have strong local governments such as counties that provide mental retardation/developmental disabilities services. This was the case in Wisconsin and Ohio. For example, Ohio has 88 county mental retardation/developmental disability boards that receive state funds to develop supported living options. Counties can: provide the supported living services themselves; advertise for what are called limited, or non-traditional, providers (that is, an agency or an individual who wants to provide discrete support services such as meal preparation, transportation and others); or contract for all supported living services from an established agency. This is a very flexible approach that can be adapted to the unique characteristics of the local area; on the other hand, with very little state control of implementation, there is significant variability regarding the quality of supported living programmes.

Organizational structures for supported living programmes were somewhat different when persons needed live-in or high levels of care and supervision. This multi-team model included an additional support person who lived with one or more individuals with mental retardation as a paid co-tenant. Typically, the in-home support workers or co-tenants had other jobs or attended school. In this model, the supported living worker is responsible for the more programmatic aspects of the service plan such as linking individuals with community resources, completing paperwork, and providing back-up support when the in-home worker is not available. Wisconsin's Options in Community Living has such a structure for individuals with severe disabilities and assigns two supported living workers to each individual receiving support (a primary worker and a back-up worker). This approach not only gives the primary worker someone else with whom to share issues and concerns, but also ensures that, when turnover occurs, the person with a disability is always with a support staff member whom they know.

Other organizational issues reflected in exemplary supported living organizations concerned the size of the agency and its commitment not only to people with disabilities but also to the staff. The executive director of Wisconsin's Options in Community Living determined that their agency would serve no more than 100 individuals with disabilities – its current size. 'My rule of thumb is that I should know every person we support personally. If that doesn't happen, we're getting too big'. Alternative Living Inc. (ALI) in Maryland came to a similar conclusion – 84 people with disabilities was the maximum number the director felt the agency could provide support to and still maintain its mission. Both agencies have been involved in creating spin-off support organizations. In 1990, three long-term staff left Options to start a new support organization called Neighbourhood Connections, which now serves about 20 people. ALI's director formed a peer support group made up of seven other agencies with the goal of 'mentoring' individuals interested in forming new organizations.

THE JOB OF BEING A SUPPORT WORKER

Staff in a supported living programme must adopt an entirely new attitude and approach towards people with disabilities. Most importantly, the support worker and the individual are on a more equal footing – the support worker works alongside the individual, not above him or her. The individual is more empowered, able to make his or her own choices (either alone or with assistance) and does not necessarily have to do whatever the support worker suggests. Indeed, one of the primary jobs of a support worker is to teach choice or decision-making. As such, the dynamics of the relationship are very different. Some supported living workers noted that they saw themselves as the individual's employee more than the agency's employee and that their primary responsibility was to serve their customers. One worker stated simply: 'What is my job? I work for Bill'.

According to several key informants, there are advantages to being support workers: greater autonomy, responsibility and opportunities for creativity; more flexibility, variability in daily activities and decentralized decision-making ('You know the person best, you decide'); and direct accountability to the individual with a disability. Support programme directors indicated they looked for support workers without preconceived notions about how to provide services and who were not afraid to 'think on their feet'. Some agencies defined the type of person they would hire as 'supported friends'.

One of the major disadvantages of being a support worker is being available 24-hours a day – in most cases, supported living staff gave their telephone numbers out to all of the individuals they supported. (In turn, this created significant incentives for staff to work with the individuals on appropriate use of the telephone.) The other disadvantage focused on the ability to remain 'engaged' or closely involved with individuals as they experimented more with lifestyle choices and control. Since supported living means giving up some level of control over people's lives, there is potential for being in a constant state of flux and moving from crisis to crisis. Crises, such as getting evicted from apartments, not getting along with roommates, choosing hazardous employment and others, are part of real life. Many support staff stressed that persons with mental retardation/developmental disabilities learn through their own successes and failures just like non-disabled people.

PAYMENT MECHANISMS AND SOURCES OF FINANCING FOR SUPPORTED LIVING

For the most part, the payment mechanisms used for supported living programmes in the five states included state contracts or grants with individual agencies or with a local unit of government (county). In Florida, some local mental retardation authorities provided cash directly to individuals for specific types of expenses: a deposit for a house, moving expenses, extraordinary medical expenses and so forth. The types of revenue streams available for supported living were highlighted earlier in the chapter. As noted in that section, four CSLA states in the study have not yet received funding targeted for the CSLA programme, and the rest of the states have either funded supported living entirely through their own resources (Florida, Ohio) or with the Medicaid Home and Community Based waiver (Wisconsin, Maryland, Illinois) together with other federal/state funds.

METHODS USED TO ENSURE THE QUALITY OF SUPPORTED LIVING SERVICES

Perhaps the thorniest issue that most observers raise with respect to implementing supported living is how to provide accountability and monitoring for a highly individualized and flexible approach to residential living. As an overall objective, it is important to stress that supported living is rooted in honouring and supporting individual choices and desires; as such, quality assurance must be individually focused. Some informants indicated that they did not want any regulation while others were afraid that government bureaucrats would regulate to the lowest common denominator.

It was commonly accepted that supported living programmes must meet some basic or minimal health and safety requirements and build in 'gentle accountability' (but not create regulatory madness). In some states, supported living regulations were very prescriptive (Illinois' standards are 52 pages long and were considered too medicalized by some informants). Florida shifted from a very prescriptive regulatory approach, including detailed housing quality standards, to a simpler, more general expression of the major goals and objectives of the supported living programme. Many informants recommended some type of person-centred planning approach as the first line of accountability in supported living.

Beyond meeting basic health and safety issues (e.g. not allowing individuals to live in filth and hazardous conditions), balancing choices with risks was addressed on an individual basis. Several respondents recommended staying with the person and 'remaining engaged' when choices lead to adverse consequences. Even the most experienced supported living agencies did not have the answers – they were continually working on helping individuals achieve a higher quality of life which, in some cases, included risks. All of these agencies stressed, however, that the rewards far outweighed the risks in supported living.

Finally, involvement of people with an independent perspective was important (e.g. through circles of support). As one key informant noted: 'If supported living is done correctly, it provides its own quality assurance – it's a self-monitoring system, especially through circles of support'. Other possible monitoring and/or evaluation mechanisms include community-wide or individually-based monitoring boards, peer review mechanisms, consumer satisfaction measurement and outcome measures such as Maryland's four questions: is the person getting the services requested/specified in his/her person-centred plan? Are they working? Is the person satisfied with the supports/services received? Do they continue to make sense with respect to the types of goals and outcomes requested or anticipated for this person?

A FUTURE RESEARCH AGENDA FOR SUPPORTED LIVING

In some ways, supported living resembles various aspects of those residential alternatives at the top of the continuum (semi-independent or supported independent living). Halpern et al. (1986) suggested that semi-independent living models should be evaluated along multiple dimensions and using a variety of research methods to reflect the complex demands of adult adjustment. These authors identified four areas of research:

- occupation and finances;
- residential environment (home, neighbourhood);
- social network;
- client satisfaction.

Consumer satisfaction is at the heart of supported living and is certainly an area in which additional evaluation can be conducted. Several analysts have also suggested that the critical outcome for supported living is improved effectiveness, that is, does a person's quality of life improve? (Ferguson et al., 1990).

Since supported living is evolving there is certainly a need to develop a research agenda that identifies both short- and long-term objectives. For example, it would be useful to assess in what ways the critical components or dimensions of supported living (e.g. choice/control, person-centred planning, control of one's home, and others) are operationalized across the United States. Are there elements of programme design and implementation that are most predictive of the successful organization and delivery of such services? (Gettings, 1992). Much of this research agenda, however, depends on getting experts in the field to agree on the defining characteristics of supported living so that a proper comparison can be made.

Gettings (1992) suggests that it is premature to conduct an outcome evaluation that asks whether supported living works and if so, for whom and why, because of the importance of potential long-term outcomes (e.g. does a supported living approach for people with challenging behaviours lead to fewer problem behaviours over time? Are individuals experiencing greater interdependence?). The focus is not on measuring skills acquisition but rather on making community connections and increasing personal satisfaction. On the other hand, there are some programmes, such as Options in Wisconsin, that have provided supported living in its purest form for over ten years and from whom outcome measures on issues such as enhanced quality of life could be taken. At the same time, it would be important to fund several observational studies of individuals participating in supported living in order to identify specific indicators to use in new measurement tools designed to capture individual change.

CONCLUSION

This chapter has provided an overview of the development of the supported living philosophy and ways in which it is being implemented in the United States. Supported living is flourishing in some parts of the country, but is still in its infancy in other areas. There is a growing disenchantment with the traditional residential continuum and what it offers individuals with their families and supported living provides possible answers for many of these individuals. It offers the potential of stretching scarce fiscal resources to meet waiting list needs, among other needs. For some individuals, there will be cost savings, while for others the costs will be greater than in traditional residential programmes. The greatest potential for achievement in a supported living approach is for individuals with mental retardation/developmental disabilities to actually participate in and become members of their local community.

Quality of support for ordinary living

8

David Felce

Recent years have seen a considerable expansion in the provision of residential services using ordinary housing for people with mental retardation, as institution closure policies have been agreed and implemented. This has been true for the United Kingdom, Scandinavia, North America and Australasia among others. Such change has been based on a critique of the negative effects of institutional regimes (e.g. Goffman, 1961; King *et al.*, 1971), the emergence and widespread influence of the principle of normalization (e.g. Bank-Mikkelsen, 1969; Nirje, 1969; Wolfensberger, 1972), legal rights to treatment and to care in the least restrictive environment (e.g. Herr, 1992) and on research which has tested the relative advantages of institutional versus community care (e.g. Allen, 1989; Conroy and Bradley, 1985; Felce *et al.*, 1980; Felce, 1989; Lowe and de Paiva 1991; Sandler and Thurman, 1981).

One of the central rationales underpinning the use of ordinary housing in the community is the desire to promote ordinary patterns of living (King's Fund, 1980; Welsh Office, 1983). The purpose of this chapter is to report the results of investigations of the characteristics of residential services which result in high resident involvement in the activities of everyday life. The research question has now moved beyond the simple comparison of large versus small, hospital or institution versus community house to a need for a closer understanding of the determinants of high quality. This may be described as progressing beyond the concentration on deinstitutionalization to a new paradigm of community membership and the concept of supported living, as Allard has argued in Chapter 7. However, it is important to ensure that staff within supported housing do actually provide support to individuals who require it and not just assume that this is what they will do. A major focus of this chapter is on the role that staff have as important mediators between, on the one hand, the opportunities inherent in ordinary housing to lead an ordinary lifestyle and, on the other, the taking up of those opportunities by individuals with severe learning disabilities who lack independence in most areas of functioning.

There is considerable scope for variation in quality among community residential services and the mere fact of a service being small and based in ordinary housing in the community is not sufficient for it to be of high quality. Tøssebro (Chapter 5) and Emerson (Chapter 11) indicate the variability of services of the same type. Many of the authors cited above have been at pains to interpret the relative advantage of community services over institutions by reference to a broad range of variables by which the evaluated services differed (e.g. Felce, 1988). As Sandler and Thurman (1981) pointed out in their review of research on the impact of deinstitutionalization on developmental progress, it is not possible to tell whether the gains made in the community services were due to the fundamental structure of the services (small size, domestic design, etc.) or to their philosophy, the training of staff, the way they operated and the extent of implementation of individualized programmes.

CLASSIFYING THE ECOLOGY OF THE RESIDENTIAL ENVIRONMENT

The scope for variation between provision which, at a broad level, could be classified as similar (e.g. institutional settings, community settings, group home settings) has prompted a number of commentators to discuss the development of a typology for community residential settings. Butler and Bjaanes (1977) suggested the distinction between custodial, therapeutic and maintaining environments. They emphasized that settings could differ in orientation although being outwardly similar. In like vein, Janicki (1981) has argued that the rehabilitative intent within the setting has to be established as a factor independent from, and one which cannot be assumed from, other setting characteristics. Interpreting our work in the Andover area of Wessex, I have suggested a three-dimensional framework for looking at the design of the service (Figure 8.1): structure, which defines the major parameters of the setting; orientation, which defines in operational terms the service's aims and therapeutic direction, and procedures, which define how staff work with residents (Felce, 1988; Felce and Repp, 1992).

Service structure, often established during the initial planning phase, is concerned with the size of the service (resident numbers), the design and furnishings of the building, whom it serves (resident groupings), where it is located, staffing numbers, roles and qualifications, the resource budget set and the extent of budgetary control devolved to the operational tier. A broad service orientation may also be set at this stage in terms of conformity to general principles or operational philosophy. Although Wolfensberger's definition and operationalization of the principle of normalization clearly extends to factors other than the structure and broad orientation of the service (e.g. Wolfensberger and Glenn, 1975), people often refer solely to structural variables when claiming that their services conform to the normalization principle. In practice, service planning rarely concerns itself with issues other than those which define service structure. However, arguably the most important dimension of service orientation is how broad principles are translated into operational policies and job descriptions, and how staff are then recruited to possess requisite skills and attitudes consistent with the aims and objectives set. This is one of the prime concerns of the managerial level of the service. Service procedures cover working methods, staff training, quality monitoring and management of staff. They are a result of managerial and operational level action. Figure 8.1 illustrates these three dimensions for an ordinary housing service similar to the one my colleagues and me established in the Andover area of Wessex, England which was designed to establish a model housing service for adults with the most severe or profound learning disabilities and produce a high level of resident development and involvement in everyday activity.

The scope for variation between services of similar structure referred to earlier is evident in the variety of factors shown in Figure 8.1 which might have an impact on outcome. For people living in staffed housing who have considerable needs for support, outcome is very much dependent on what staff do. In understanding how to provide effective support for ordinary living within services, we need to distinguish what level and quality of staff:resident interaction promotes resident participation and independence. We then need to look at what service design features, in terms of procedural, orientational and structural variables, may account for such staff and resident activity. What follows is an exploration of these two related questions using two databases: the first is from the research already referred to undertaken in Andover in the 1980s and the second is a more recent survey of housing services in South Wales done this decade. The remainder of the chapter is structured in four sections:

- a brief review of the literature on staff:resident interaction and resident participation in activity;
- a summary of the staff and resident activity data from the Andover research;
- a summary of the staff and resident activity data from the housing services in South Wales;
- an interpretation of the comparative results.

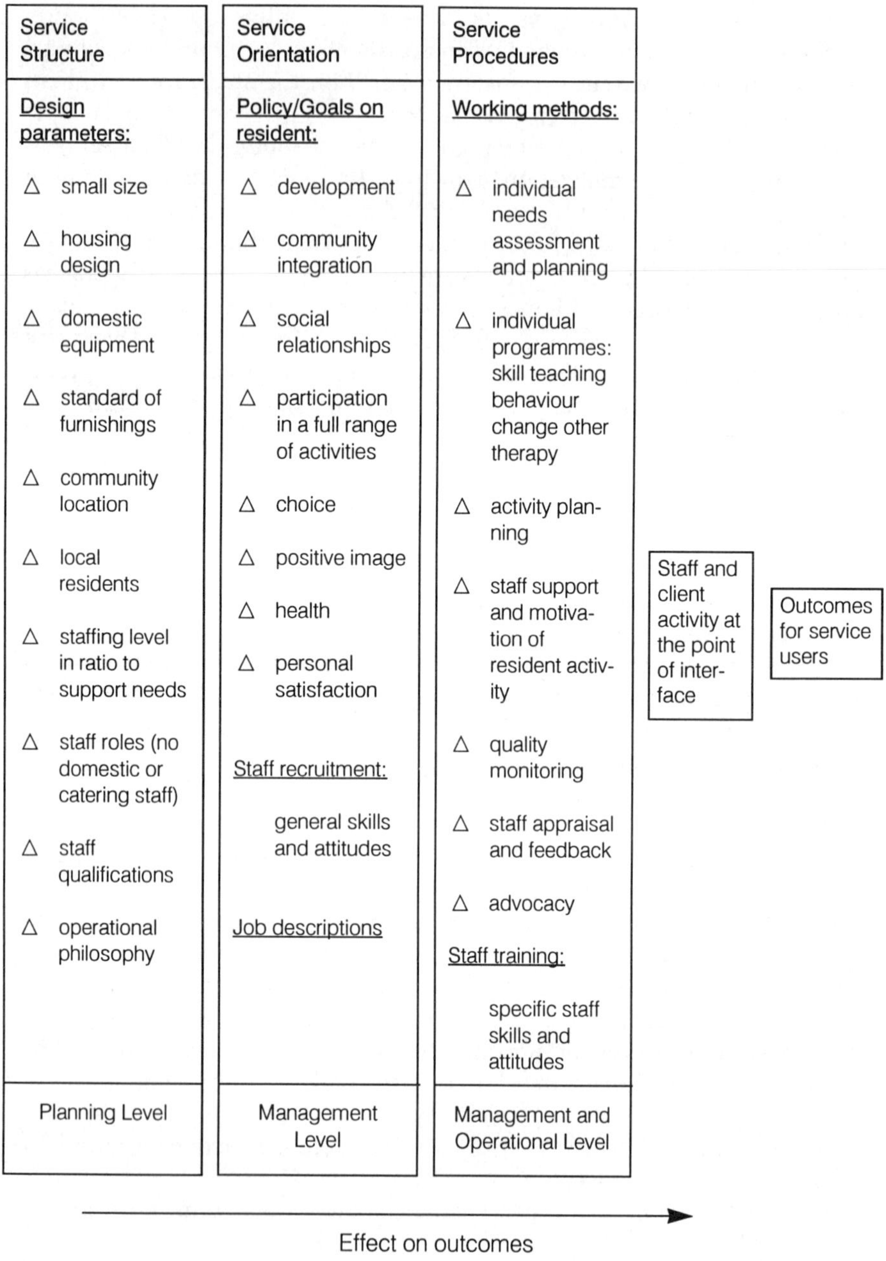

Service Structure	Service Orientation	Service Procedures
Design parameters:	Policy/Goals on resident:	Working methods:
△ small size	△ development	△ individual needs assessment and planning
△ housing design	△ community integration	
△ domestic equipment	△ social relationships	△ individual programmes: skill teaching behaviour change other therapy
△ standard of furnishings	△ participation in a full range of activities	
△ community location	△ choice	△ activity planning
△ local residents	△ positive image	△ staff support and motivation of resident activity
△ staffing level in ratio to support needs	△ health	
	△ personal satisfaction	
△ staff roles (no domestic or catering staff)	Staff recruitment:	△ quality monitoring
△ staff qualifications	general skills and attitudes	△ staff appraisal and feedback
		△ advocacy
△ operational philosophy	Job descriptions	Staff training:
		specific staff skills and attitudes
Planning Level	Management Level	Management and Operational Level

Staff and client activity at the point of interface

Outcomes for service users

→ Effect on outcomes

Figure 8.1 Design framework for staffed ordinary housing.

STAFFING, RESIDENT DEPENDENCY, STAFF PERFORMANCE AND RESIDENT PARTICIPATION IN ACTIVITY

As severity of disability or dependency on others increases, the need for more intense and consistent support increases, if the goal of achieving ordinary patterns of activity is to be maintained. Therefore, it is logical to expect that the staffing level within ordinary housing schemes will be higher in services which cater for people with greater dependency. Associated expectations are that increased staffing will be reflected in a greater level of staff support directed towards residents, and that increased staff input will provide an effective bridge for residents to engage in activities despite their limited independent abilities. However, many observational studies of institutional settings have shown extremely low rates of interaction between staff and residents, at levels clearly insufficient for people who need support to do the majority of personal and household activities involved in ordinary homelife (e.g. Burg *et al.*, 1979; Cullen *et al.*, 1983; Landesman-Dwyer *et al.*, 1980; Moores and Grant, 1976; Oswin, 1978; Rawlings, 1985; Wood, 1989; Wright *et al.*, 1974). According to this research, individuals can expect contact from staff only a few times per hour for less than a minute on each occasion.

Landesman (1988) has described the lack of sufficient social interaction with residents as 'the primary fault in the behaviour of direct care staff'. She has also suggested that the overwhelming belief among most service personnel that this low amount of interaction is due to staff shortage should be called the myth of understaffing. Landesman-Dwyer *et al.* (1980) found that staff:resident ratios were not correlated with staff:resident interaction rates across a number of large group homes. Moreover, studies in a range of different types of facility have found that increases in staff have not necessarily been accompanied by proportional increases in staff interaction with residents (Duker *et al.*., 1991; Felce *et al.*, 1991; Harris *et al.*, 1974; Mansell *et al.*, 1982; Seys and Duker, 1988). For example, the first study cited showed that staff spent more time engaged in organizational duties and less time providing stimulation to residents when there were greater rather than lower average levels of staff on duty.

Despite the fact that people with more severe or profound learning disabilities require more support from staff, observational research does not show that they differentially receive more interaction from staff. Residents with lower levels of independence, adaptive behaviour or intellectual competence have been found to receive less positive interactions, informative speech, or attention than their more able counterparts (e.g. Dailey *et al.*, 1974; Grant and Moores, 1977; Pratt *et al.*, 1976). Duker *et al.* (1989) demonstrated that resident behaviour influences the frequency of resident directed initiatives from staff, with those who are more alert and likely to interact with staff receiving more staff contact. They also found, on the one hand, positive relationships between adaptive behaviour and levels of training and staff stimulation, and on the other, an inverse relationship between adaptive behaviour and receipt of custodial care. Those with greater disabilities, therefore, received fewer staff-initiated interactions, less training and stimulation and more routine custodial care.

A second theme underlying staff allocation policies is the presumption that staff would, in their interaction, act to support residents to be involved in typical daily living activities. However, when staff do interact with residents, it is often in a way which is not intended to promote resident engagement in activity. Staff in institutions have been shown to spend a low proportion of their time in training activities and to give very little direct instruction, prompting or physical assistance to residents (e.g. Felce *et al.*, 1986; Moores and Grant, 1976; Seys and Duker, 1988; Wood, 1989). Rather, the great majority of their interaction has been found to be in the form of general conversation and other forms of 'neutral' contact (i.e. with no apparent purpose to encourage or discourage any form of resident behaviour). In a study which particularly sought to investigate whether staff chose to employ the forms of interaction which were most likely to help residents engage successfully in activities, Repp *et al.* (1982) found that staff rarely used the form of instruction most likely to help residents respond correctly (non-verbal instruction either with or without physical assistance) and usually employed the form of instruction (verbal instruction) which most likely led to non-response.

In summary, there are a number of points of possible breakdown in the linkage between high staff numbers, extensive staff interaction with residents and high resident participation in the daily living concerns which occupy us all. One possibility is that such problems as the lack of resident activity and the low level of staff support given to residents are features purely of institutional structures and regimes. A belief that service structures alone are sufficient to determine quality of outcome would lead to the expectation that such deficiencies are less likely to occur in small, more normalized settings in the community. Already, such a proposition is in doubt as can be judged from the title of a book chapter by Landesman (1988) referring to 'preventing institutionalisation in the community'. Research is, therefore, required to establish the factors which guarantee quality.

RESEARCH ON STAFF:RESIDENT INTERACTION AND RESIDENT PARTICIPATION IN ACTIVITY IN ANDOVER

It is not my intention here to describe this body of research in detail as it has been published for some time (Felce, 1988; 1989; 1991; Felce and Repp, 1992 for summary overviews and further references). Rather, I want to draw out a number of results from various studies which are relevant to the interpretation of the quality of staff and resident activity and to present a new analysis of the interrelationship between resident activity, staff interaction with residents and resident abilities. In this and the later work in Wales, resident abilities were measured using the Adaptive Behavior Scale (ABS) (Nihira *et al.*, 1974), a total score being derived by summing across all domains with the exception of the vocational domain which was omitted. Resident and staff activity were observed directly using the Activity Measure (Beasley, Hewson and Mansell, 1989; Mansell *et al.*, 1984). Readers are referred to the papers cited for precise details of observational definitions, procedures and the reliability of the data.

Felce *et al.* (1986) produced data on resident engagement in personal (self-care), leisure, domestic and social activities and the extent and nature of staff interactions with residents in the first two Andover houses. Six residents in each group had mean total ABS scores of 117 and 105 but ability groupings reflected a degree of heterogeneity (ranges, 62–168 and 54–143). Staff:resident ratios averaged 1:2.4 and 1:2.2 in Houses 1 and 2 respectively. On average, each resident received interaction from staff for 27% and 20% of time respectively of which nearly 80% was in the form of instruction, demonstration and physical prompting or assistance to do an activity (22% and 14% of time for each resident in each house on average). Residents were engaged in non-social activity (personal, leisure and domestic activities) for 51% and 56% of time on average and social activity (mainly with staff) for 17% and 14%. The majority of these data are depicted as part of Figures 8.2 and 8.3.

The relationships between staff support and resident dependency and between staff support and resident activity concealed within the above averages are interesting. Unlike much previous research, individuals with greater disabilities received more support from staff (defined in terms of receipt of instruction, demonstration, prompting and guidance). There was a perfect inverse relationship between total ABS score and the amount of support received from staff among the first group of six residents and a Spearman rank order correlation coefficient of –0.77 among the second group (and an overall r_s = –0.76, p<0.01). Moreover, as we had two sets of observations on most subjects, we could explore the correlation between the differences in support given to each resident and the differences in their level of engagement in activity. A Spearman rank order correlation coefficient on these within-subject differences was near perfect (r_s = 0.97, p<0.01). Visual inspection of the individual resident activity data suggested that the impact of high levels of staff support for those with greater disabilities was to bring their levels of engagement in activity up towards those of the more able.

Such findings suggest that resident activity in these houses could be expressed as a function of resident ability and the extent of staff support (i.e. residents brought something to the service in terms of their abilities to do various activities and staff added to this by supporting residents to be more involved than they might otherwise have been able). This analysis was not pursued at the time but I have recently undertaken it using a two-stage linear regression model. Multivariate regression was unsatisfactory due to the high negative correlation between resident ability and staff support (Pearson's $r = -0.66$). Therefore, the relationship between the level of resident engagement in activity and staff support was estimated first, controlling for ability, by regressing the within-subject differences in engagement level across pairs of data points against similar differences in staff support. This produced a linear function to predict the level of activity attributable to staff support. This function produced an adjusted R Square of 0.82 (i.e. it explained 82% of the variance in the dependent variable) and an F ratio which was significant at 0.0002. The level of engagement not attributable to staff support was then calculated by deducting the engagement explained by the above function from the average level of engagement found for each subject. This residual engagement level was then regressed in the second stage of the analysis against resident ability in the form of ABS scores converted to average percentile ranks. This second function also produced a satisfactory function with an adjusted R Square of 0.72 (i.e. ability explained 72% of the variance of residual engagement) and an F ratio significant at 0.001.

In summary, the analysis of the data from this study strongly suggests that the extent of staff support (i.e. the extent and nature of staff:resident interaction) was important in determining the extent of resident engagement in activity. The first part of the two-stage linear regression describes the 'value-added' especially to residents with greater disabilities by the presence and activity of staff. The second part shows the contribution of the resident's own skills to outcome.

Two further data sets collected on staff:resident interaction and resident activity in these and other similar houses emphasize other aspects of the social ecology worthy of mention here. Felce et al. (1987) explored the contingency of staff attention on resident behaviour. When residents were appropriately engaged (as opposed to being passive, having nothing to do or behaving inappropriately), they were likely to receive attention from staff within 15 seconds 57% of the time (compared to 33% and 34% for residents in institutions or large community units). Moreover, 77% of staff attention was given to residents when they were appropriately engaged (compared to 51% and 69% in institutions and large community units). Contingency of attention on engagement in activity has been shown to increase the level of activity (Porterfield *et al.*, 1980; Mansell, Felce, de Kock *et al.*, 1982). Therefore, the level of engagement in the houses can be said to owe something to the motivational climate established by staff when they attended to residents.

Felce *et al.* (1991) investigated the extent of both staff:resident interaction and resident engagement in activity as a function of size of staff:resident group. Arithmetically identical staff:resident ratios did not produce similar activity patterns. For example, in every case the larger staff:resident group was associated with lower resident activity. In general across institutional, large community unit, and ordinary housing settings, an effective return from increasing staff was found when staff were assigned to work individually with smaller resident groups but not when more staff were allocated to larger resident groups, a result consistent with other findings (e.g. Harris *et al.*, 1974; Orlowska *et al.*, 1991).

The above studies suggest that the resident activity found in the Andover houses results from a combination of factors, with staff support and motivation central to the analysis. The interpretation which appears to fit the data which I have advanced (Felce, 1989) based on the service design framework offered in Figure 8.1 is summarized by three sets of relationships set out in Figure 8.4: the supportive model, the motivational model and the organizational model. The supportive model relates to the emphasis on instruction, demonstration, prompting and guidance within the approach staff took to helping residents with very substantial disabilities to be involved in the routine aspects of their daily household lives. Such staff performance does not occur in a vacuum and needs to be present or reflected in service orientation, structure and procedures. In the Andover service, an emphasis on resident engagement in activity was central to orientation, not just in relation to those activities for which residents possessed or nearly possessed the skills but to all activities necessary for everyday life. This was set down in detail in the service's operational policy and staff job descriptions (Mansell *et al.*, 1987). Ordinary activity requires the pre-conditions of an ordinary environmental context: a decent material environment and full access by residents, irrespective of level of disability, to the functional areas of the home, such as kitchen and utility area. Finally, on the basis that much other research would suggest that this supportive mode of interaction is not generally reached by intuition, staff were given training on how to interact to provide sufficient help for residents to participate in all activities rather than having things done to or for them.

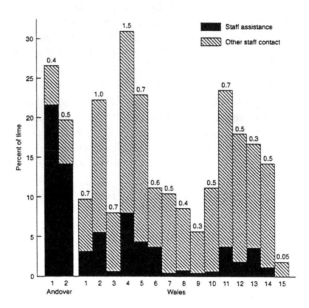

Figure 8.2 Total staff contact and staff assistance (instruction and physical guidance) per resident (with numbers of staff per resident).

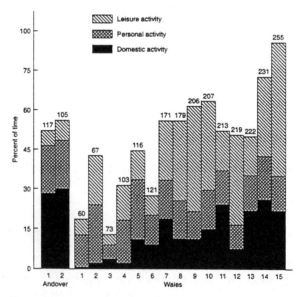

Figure 8.3 Engagement in non-social activity in 17 houses (with average total ABS scores on top of each histogram).

The motivational model refers to frequent attention being given to residents when appropriately engaged in activity. Again staff were given training on the importance of their attention as a motivational force and, therefore, when to interact with residents. However, establishing resident engagement via the supportive model appears to be a pre-requisite of the motivational model. Without the supportive model, residents with the most severe or profound disabilities will infrequently engage in activity appropriately (e.g. the 'low engagers' group in the study by Mansell, Felce, de Kock *et al.*, 1982). Giving them attention at times other than when they are passive, disengaged or behaving inappropriately is made more difficult or virtually impossible as a result. (Staff in the institutional settings studied where the supportive model was not in place gave half of their attention to residents when they were passive, disengaged or behaving inappropriately. No differential motivation of appropriate engagement was, therefore, established.)

The organizational model highlights practical systems by which staff plan and monitor the opportunities and support they offer residents to be involved in activity throughout the day. Staff deployment and staff:resident activity groupings were not left to chance in the Andover houses. A planning system was operated by each oncoming staff shift every day in which they worked out who was to do what, where and with whom during their period on duty. Opportunities actually made available to each resident were recorded at the end of the shift and summarized to inform the regular weekly review of what was being achieved. The creation of small staff:resident groups which were found to be conducive to activity is supported by the small size of the service. The design of ordinary housing (with its typical variety and function of rooms) may also help divide the overall staff and resident group into several one-to-one or one-to-small-group working units.

In summary, staff interaction with residents and resident activity are interconnected and depend on the interaction of factors within the orientation, structure and procedures of the service. The Andover houses followed working methods which resulted in staff planning their responsibilities for the conduct of a range of ordinary household activities with individuals or small resident groups. The training given to staff on how to interact to support and motivate residents provided them with a practical way of succeeding in involving residents with substantial disabilities in functional tasks. An equally practical way of monitoring achievement reinforced the orientation set and allowed revision of what was being accomplished. I believe that the results of our research on the Andover houses did not show that they were better than the other services we compared them against because they were small, ordinary

The Supportive Model	Staff provide extensive assistance to individuals with substantial disabilities (instruction, demonstration, prompting and guidance)	
Service Design Pre-requisites		
Orientation	**Structure**	**Procedures**
Engagement as key part of operational policy	Ordinary environmental context	Access to functional everyday activities
Staff role to support engagement written into job descriptions	Access to functional everyday activities	Training in staff support strategies:
Veto on care and 'hotel' models		Instruct/Show/ Prompt/Guide

The Motivational Model	Staff provide frequent attention contingent on resident engagement	
Service Design Pre-requisites		
Orientation	**Structure**	**Procedures**
Engagement as key part of operational policy	Ordinary environmental context	Training in staff motivation strategies:
Staff role to motivate engagement written into job description	Access to functional everyday activities	Contingent attention
Veto on care and 'hotel' models		Operation of the Supportive Model

The Organizational Model	Planned activities and staff deployment Planned small staff: resident groupings Monitoring of activity opportunities Feedback to staff	
Service Design Pre-requisites		
Orientation	**Structure**	**Procedures**
Engagement as key part of operational policy	Ordinary environmental context	Planning and Monitoring systems:
Staff role to support engagement written into job descriptions	Small size	to cover staff and resident activity throughout the day
Veto on care and 'hotel' models	Ordinary house design	

Figure 8.4 The supportive, motivational and organizational models to promote resident engagement.

houses, or even small, ordinary, well-staffed houses in the community, but because these attributes were coupled with a well-operationalized orientation and a set of working procedures and staff training methods to match.

RESEARCH ON STAFF:RESIDENT INTERACTION AND RESIDENT PARTICIPATION IN ACTIVITY IN SOUTH WALES

Evaluation of some more recently provided staffed housing schemes (in England: Bratt and Johnston, 1988; Hewson and Walker, 1992; and Ireland: Conneally *et al.*, 1992) supports the conclusion from the Andover research that the beneficial staff and resident activity were a consequence not only of the changed service structure but also of the working methods and training adopted. Bratt and Johnston (1988) referred to subsequent new staffed housing projects as 'second generation' services to indicate that they had been provided by ordinary service authorities in the wake of 'model' research developments. They suggested that evaluation of these services was important as it was quite possible that they would be provided without the same attention to procedural detail as the first well-researched examples. Their own study showed that outcome in such services could compare poorly to results from research demonstration projects; they concluded that 'there was little or no evidence (in the services they looked at) of individuals being supported in ways that increased their competence'. Hewson and Walker (1992) showed that staff in 11 community homes interacted with residents at levels comparable to those in the services evaluated in Andover. However, in contrast to the findings of Felce, de Kock and Repp (1986), 80% of the staff:resident interaction in these houses was 'neutral' (i.e. was not directed at promoting resident participation in activity); less than 10% of the staff contact given to residents in half of the houses being in the form of direct assistance with activities. Conneally *et al.* (1992) provided data on resident engagement and staff:resident interaction in two group homes, which they argued confirmed the advantage of small, homely environments. However, they showed that engagement levels improved within the homes over time, particularly in one of the houses, as staff gave more assistance to residents as a result of training. This finding supports the contention that training and working methods are important and that high quality staff activity may not be an automatic feature of ordinary housing services.

One of the aims of the research in South Wales was, therefore, to see whether recently provided staffed housing services developed under the auspices of the All Wales Mental Handicap Strategy (Welsh Office, 1983) to encourage ordinary patterns of living were, in fact, doing that to the maximum extent possible. Considerable emphasis has been given by the Welsh Office to ensuring that schemes funded under the Strategy conformed to the small ordinary house model (Beyer *et al.*, 1991). Funding has often been generous so that services can have the advantage of high staffing levels. However, Welsh Office influence on service quality through their concern for the size of the service and the nature and location of the service setting, and through their preparedness to fund advantageous staff:resident ratios has been limited, according to the analysis set out above, to structural variables. As I have argued, the variables may indeed be important but not precisely linked to outcome in the absence of more close attention being given to service orientation and procedures. The housing services in Wales were 'second-generation' in the Bratt and Johnston (1988) sense in being provided by a variety of ordinary local authority, health authority or private and voluntary agencies, with operational policies, staff training and working methods determined locally.

Fifteen houses were selected to reflect a range of dependency levels. All served adults and ranged in size from one to seven places. The houses catered for a total of 57 residents at the outset of the study. The houses are numbered in Figures 8.2 and 8.3 in order of ascending total ABS score. In general, ability groupings within houses were homogenous. Residents in Houses 1–3 had domain profiles typical of the lowest quartile of people in the large American sample from which the ABS reference norms were derived. Low proportions possessed basic self-help skills such as continence or the abilities to feed, dress and wash; the ability to speak in sentences was virtually absent. Residents of Houses 4, 5 and 6 had greater self-help skills than those in the first three houses. However, they too had little spoken language. Residents in Houses 7–15 generally had good self-help skills and could speak in sentences. Higher proportions had literacy skills in the higher numbered houses. Residents in houses 13, 14 and 15 had ABS domain profiles typical of the upper quartile of the American reference sample.

Figure 8.2 shows the percentage of time each resident, on average, received contact from staff and the nature of that attention in terms of either assistance to do an activity or another type of contact. It also shows the level of staffing in terms of numbers of staff on duty per resident. Total interaction from staff received per resident was variable across the 15 Welsh houses, with a mean extent of 15% of time per person (range, 2%–31%). The variability in staff interaction with residents was not greatly related to resident dependency. Slightly higher levels of interaction per resident were found in the first six houses serving the most disabled residents (mean, 18%) compared to the higher numbered nine houses (mean, 12%). But overall, there was a small, non-significant inverse Spearman rank order correlation between interaction per resident and resident ability($r_s = -0.11$). The slightly higher rates of interaction received per resident in the houses for those with the greatest disabilities were the result of considerably higher staffing levels. When the staff:resident ratio is taken into account it is clear that, in common with research cited in the literature review, staff in the Welsh houses for more able people interacted more with residents than those in the lower numbered houses (mean interaction per staff: 20% of time in Houses 1–6 and 32% in Houses 7–15).

The average proportion of the total staff interaction with residents which was given in the form of assistance to do activities was 15% (range, 0%–35%). Each resident on average received assistance for 2.5% of time (means across houses ranged from 0%–8%). Residents in Houses 1–6 received greater assistance, on average for 4.2% of time, compared to 1.4% for residents in Houses 7–15. However, overall the inverse correlation between level of assistance and resident ability was not significant ($r_s = -0.41$). Moreover, even in Houses 1–6, the most disabled residents, many with ABS scores in the bottom quartile of the range, received assistance for only one minute in 25.

In comparison to the level of staff:resident interaction in the Andover houses also shown in Figure 8. 2 and discussed earlier, a number of differences are found with respect to the Welsh houses. There was less interaction per resident found in most Welsh houses. When staff:resident ratios are taken into account the comparison is made more stark. The four Welsh houses with similar or higher staff interaction per resident compared to the Andover houses (Houses 2, 4, 5 and 11) had staff:resident ratios 75%–375% higher. Six houses (1, 3, 6, 7, 8, 10) with similar or up to 75% higher staff:resident ratios produced only half the Andover level of staff interaction per resident. Two houses (12 and 13) produced similar levels of staff interaction with residents with approximately similar staff:resident ratios. These comparisons are emphasized by looking at the percentage time spent interacting with residents by each staff, calculated by multiplying the staff:resident interaction per resident by the number of residents per staff. The average in the two Andover houses (55%, range, 44%–65%) was twice that in the 15 Welsh houses (27%). The percentage of time staff spent interacting with residents varied greatly between the Welsh houses, a more than fivefold difference between lowest and highest (range, 12%–65%). Further, the proportion of staff interaction in the form of assistance was 70% and 81% in the two Andover houses but only 15% on average in the Welsh houses. The highest proportion (35%, found in House 6) was half that found in the Andover houses. There are clearly very great differences in the extent of support for ordinary living occurring within different ordinary housing services.

Figure 8.3 shows data on the engagement of residents in day-to-day activity within the houses, together with the average total ABS scores of house residents. Engagement in activity varied sixfold across the Welsh houses (range, 13%–88%) and averaged 49%. Variation was significantly related to resident ability ($r_s = 0.79$, p<0.01). Engagement in non-social engagement depicted in Figure 8.3 excludes engagement in social interaction by residents with staff or other residents. This particularly occurred in Houses 11, 12 and 13, which had a lower level of engagement in non-social activity than is suggested by the rising trend of the data across ability levels. Had total engagement in social and non-social activity been considered, the relationship between engagement and ability would be shown to be even stronger ($r_s = 0.90$). Average total engagement across all Welsh houses was 54%. Engagement in personal activity (mainly eating and drinking) was relatively constant across houses. Participation in running their own households as evidenced by engagement in domestic activity was virtually non-existent for residents in Houses 1–4 and rose to levels around 25% of the time for residents in Houses 13–15. Engagement in domestic activity overall averaged 13% of time and was significantly related to resident ability ($r_s = 0.84$, p<0.01). Engagement in leisure activity also tended to rise with ability; it was the largest component of activity in the majority of Houses 7–15. Much comprised fairly passive activity such as watching television (an activity defined as 'neutral' rather than engaged in the Andover research).

Engagement in activity in the Andover houses was above that in Wales for people of similar dependency (Houses 4–6) and similar to that for residents of much greater ability (Houses 7–13). Participation in household activities among Andover residents was greater than the highest in any of the Welsh houses, twice the average level and four times any level in Houses 1–6. As has been discussed above, the scale of staff support given to Andover house residents was not found in Wales. Welsh resident engagement in activity was primarily a function of their ability and this was particularly manifested in low engagement in household activities, particularly in the lower numbered houses.

INTERPRETATION AND CONCLUSIONS

Findings from South Wales are consistent with the earlier interpretation of the Andover research as set against the research literature: staff:resident interaction and resident engagement in activity are a function not only of structural variables but also of orientation and working methods. In many ways, the Welsh houses would be seen as better than the Andover houses in terms of service structure. They were more recently provided at a time when a more general acceptance of the ordinary life philosophy had been achieved in comparison with a decade earlier. They were, on the whole, smaller in size and better staffed. However, all of the houses had less well-operationalized policies and less well-defined outcome targets. None had any systematic approach to how staff should work with residents to support and motivate particular patterns of activity. None had any well-developed methods for activity planning or working out staff:resident deployment. Moreover, apart from relatively recent and sometimes fragile attempts in some of the houses to instigate a system of individual plan review, there was little evidence of individual assessment or the implementation of teaching or behavioural development programmes.

The Welsh housing data compared to the earlier Andover benchmark emphasize the conclusion that what happens at the interface between staff and residents together with the resulting pattern of resident activity is dependent not only on the structure of the service but its detailed orientation, procedures, staff training and management practices. The Welsh houses were less well-developed in these latter respects than the Andover services and the staff:resident interaction and resident engagement data were poorer despite equivalent or more advantageous service structures. The pursuit of quality in ordinary housing services entails more than just the provision of ordinary environments.

Such a pursuit involves changing performance away from traditional care or 'hotel' models (where staff relieve residents of all responsibility for household management as if staying in a hotel) and creating an alternative which emphasizes resident participation. It also involves changing performance away from the traditional allocation of activity to residents, on the basis of their ability to carry out activities independently and creating an alternative which emphasizes the absence of exclusion of residents from participation and the provision of support to help those people who lack skills to accomplish activity successfully. It also involves changing performance away from the traditional *laissez-faire* attitude to what activities residents may or may not do and creating an alternative which gives positive motivation to achieving that level of functional activity which everyone else needs to achieve to live an ordinary life. Finally, it involves changing performance away from the traditional low emphasis on the organization of opportunities to participate in activity and to receive individualized instruction and behavioural or treatment programmes and creating an alternative which establishes a level of commitment, staff competence and managerial monitoring to ensure that these happen.

ACKNOWLEDGEMENTS

This research was conducted under a grant from the Welsh Office/Department of Health. We are grateful for the cooperation of the services and service users involved.

PART THREE:

The Impact on Service Users

Immediate psychological effects of deinstitutionalization

9

Timo Saloviita

During the last 20 years numerous studies have evaluated the effects of deinstitutionalization on the lives of people with intellectual disabilities. Recent reviews of these studies show typically long lists of various measures which all indicate the superiority of community living arrangements compared to traditional institutions (Haney, 1988; Larson and Lakin, 1991; Rotegard *et al.*, 1985). Most people in the field today are ready to affirm the supremacy of community living compared to institutions with regard to environmental quality and development of personal independence and quality of life. An effective summary of this debate is given by Conroy and Feinstein (1990), who state:

> Although it is theoretically possible to construct a community service system that produces worse results than the institutional model, it must be very hard to do so; otherwise, it would have been done by now, and someone would have documented it.
>
> (Conroy and Feinstein, 1990)

The successful outcome of community-based arrangements does not mean that the process of moving into the community is unproblematic. For example, parents of children with disabilities have expressed many doubts concerning this process (Larson and Lakin, 1991; Chapters 13, 14 and 15). Many of these doubts express real problems associated with transition into the community and living in it.

Heller (1982) surveyed 187 people after their developmentally disabled relatives had been transferred from an institution into the community. People with the greatest closure-related stress were those with worries about transfer trauma and those who had experienced high stress upon initial diagnosis and placement of their relatives. Family dissatisfaction was correlated with worries about transfer trauma and meeting their relatives' medical needs. In Sweden Tuvesson (Chapter 13) interviewed parents about their worries around deinstitutionalization. The three groups of worries expressed by parents were the fear of instability of the new placement, lack of services in the new residence, and fears concerning the trauma of relocation.

In a recent Finnish study 50 parents were asked about their doubts and worries concerning the move of their intellectually disabled child from an institution into the community (Saloviita, 1992). The most common doubt, expressed by 47% of parents, was suspicion about the stability of the new living arrangement. After this (35%) came the worry about adjustment of the child to the new environment after life in an institution. It was only after these questions that concern about the adequacy of various supports in community settings was expressed (Saloviita, 1992).

This concern about the stressfulness of deinstitutionalization is thus commonly expressed by parents. That it is a realistic and appropriate concern is shown by studies indicating various negative consequences associated with transfer, especially in the gerontological literature, where it is referred to as relocation syndrome or transfer trauma. Expressions of transfer trauma vary from increased mortality rates of elderly residents from nursing homes (Aldrich and Mendkoff, 1963) or psychiatric hospitals (Saathoff *et al.*, 1992) to adverse physical health effects and various negative emotional, behavioural and mental health changes (Heller, 1984).

RESEARCH WITH INTELLECTUALLY DISABLED PEOPLE

Because the phenomenon of transfer trauma is usually temporary, the most interesting studies are those which include some follow-up measurements within the first month after the move. Unfortunately, follow-up studies typically have used longer periods for data collection points and, therefore, only a few outcome studies with intellectually disabled subjects are available. In addition, recent studies on this theme seem to be lacking. Table 9.1 summarizes results from those few studies available and even among these, three follow-up points have been applied which are longer than one month. Apart from these studies there are two reviews by Heller (1984; 1988).

The results of these studies demonstrate the presence of various forms of transfer trauma among persons with intellectual disabilities who have moved from an institution into community services. The reported forms of transfer trauma include increase in maladaptive behaviour, decrease of adaptive behaviour, health problems and emotional problems. The manifestations of transfer trauma typically are of short duration – usually only a few weeks. In the long run the reported outcomes of a move have been positive. The effect of transfer appears to depend on the level of mental retardation. Lastly, no signs of transfer trauma were observed in the one study that applied a preparatory programme prior to the move.

The question of transfer trauma among persons with intellectual disabilities is important in two ways. Firstly, the observation of immediate, short-term, negative effects is possibly the only negative consequence documented concerning the deinstitutionalization process. Secondly, the worry about transfer trauma has a high priority among parents and may be an important reason for parental opposition towards the closure of institutions.

Even if the prospect of transfer trauma does prompt some parents to oppose the move of their relative into the community, the risk of transfer trauma should not be used to argue against care in the community. The community placement of people with intellectual disabilities is seen increasingly as a human right and not as a question in need of empirical verification. The question, then, is to find ways to prevent or minimize the manifestations of transfer trauma during the move to the community.

FACTORS INFLUENCING TRANSFER TRAUMA

In order to better understand the data presented it is necessary to look at the current understanding of the phenomenon of transfer trauma. Because there are so few studies on the theme made with intellectually disabled people, findings from the gerontological research are also valuable.

Transfer trauma is mostly discussed in the context of the theory of stress. Lazarus and Folkman (1984, p.19) define psychological stress as a 'particular relationship between the person and the environment that is appraised by the person as taxing or exceeding his or her resources and endangering his or her well-being'. They present two mediating processes in the person–environment relationship: cognitive appraisal and coping. Through cognitive appraisal the person evaluates and re-evaluates the significance of what is happening. Lazarus and Folkman define coping as constantly changing cognitive and behavioural efforts to manage demands that are appraised as stressful. Closely resembling this analysis Schulz and Brenner (1977) presented two related factors mediating the response to stress: controllability and predictability. They offered the following hypotheses:

- The greater the choice the individual has, the less negative the effects of relocation.

Table 9.1 Studies of transfer trauma among intellectually disabled people who have moved from institutions to the community

Name	Subjects	Method of assessment	Time of measurement	Preparatory programme	Manifestations of 'relocation syndrome'
Cochran, Sran and Varano (1977)	5 adults with mental retardation or schizophrenia	Case study	From arrival to 1 month	Not reported	Depression (5), pneumonia (2), weight loss (4), death (1). Recovery within 1 month
Cohen et al. (1977)	66 subjects with mental retardation	AAMD AB Scale	Before departure, 1–2 weeks post-exit 6–8 weeks post-exit	Not reported	High functioning: lowered functioning and withdrawal. Low functioning: increased maladaptive behaviour. Recovery within 1–2 months
Heller (1982)	50 children with severe or profound mental retardation	Observation and Fairview Development Scale	Before departure, 2 weeks post-exit 4–6 weeks post-exit 11–13 weeks post-exit	Not reported	Decrements in positive behaviour and deterioration in health. Recovery within 1 month
Hemming, Lavender and Pill (1981)	50 adults with severe mental retardation	AAMD AB Scale	Before departure, 4 months post-exit 9 months post-exit	Not reported	Increase in maladaptive behaviour at 4 months. Recovery at 9 months

Kleinberg and Galligan (1983)	20 adults with profound to moderate mental retardation	AAMD AB Scale Minnesota Developmental Programming System	Before departure, 4 months post-exit 8 months post-exit 12 months post-exit	Not reported	Antisocial behaviour increased in the group of profound retardation
O'Neill et al. (1985)	27 adults with severe or profound mental retardation	Activity Pattern and Skill Indicator	Before departure, 3 months post-exit 9 months post-exit	Not reported	No negative changes
Weinstock et al. (1979)	22 adults with profound to mild mental retardation, 22 matched controls	PAC Chart AAMD AB Scale Part Two	Before departure, 1 week post-exit 2 weeks post-exit 4 weeks post-exit	Yes	No negative changes

- The more predictable a new environment is, the less negative the effects of relocation.
- To the extent that relocation results in a decline in the controllability of the environment, the individual should be affected negatively by the move.

PREPARATORY PROGRAMMES

The ideas obtained from research on stress have been used to plan preparatory programmes for those people who are moving in order to make their move more predictable and controllable. Many studies which have included preparatory programmes have reported no signs of transfer trauma. This is true for the elderly (Jasnau, 1967; Novick, 1967; Zweig and Csank, 1975), those with intellectual disabilities (Weinstock et al., 1979), and psychiatric patients (Lentz and Paul, 1971). The study by Lentz and Paul (1971) with psychiatric patients is especially interesting because they used a control group. The experimental group, which was prepared to move, exhibited no negative effects, whereas the functional level of the control group decreased. This difference was observable one month after the move but it had disappeared after six months. The preparatory programme consisted of delivery of information about the new place and visits to it. Any anxiety expressed was responded to by reassurance and the provision of information.

SOCIAL SUPPORT

Coffman (1981) carried out a meta-analysis of data concerning 26 relocated groups of elderly people. He found no general relocation effect and no systematic effect of age, sex, mental or physical status, choice, preparation, environmental change, or mass versus individualized transfer on post-move mortality. Instead Coffman (1981) found clear mortality differences between two types of relocation processes, which he called integrative and disintegrative. By disintegrative processes Coffman (1981) meant the serious deterioration in the support systems – either actual or perceived aspects of support. He hypothesized that when the loss of support is faster and greater than its replacement, the predominant process is disintegrative and potentially harmful. When replacement support is promptly and abundantly available, the overall process is integrative and potentially beneficial. Typically, the removal process was integrative when a whole institutional or ward population was moved or when individuals moved from one stable population to another. The process was disintegrative when a whole institution was closed down or its members were redistributed.

The importance of social support was documented in a study by Wells and Macdonald (1981). They analysed the expressions of transfer trauma among 56 elderly residents who moved from an old institution that was closed down. The home was phased out over four months with transfers of residents and staff occurring throughout this period. Usually, two to four residents were moved at a time. A special programme was developed to prepare them through the relocation. The goals of this programme were to provide support and information, deal with emotional distress, and enhance autonomy and self-esteem. The subjects were followed up 8–12 weeks after they were relocated. The results showed that the relocation contributed to mental disorganization, confusion, apathy and behavioural deterioration of the residents. This happened despite the preparatory programme. However, the existence of close primary relationships with staff and ties outside the home were associated with successful adjustment to relocation in terms of life satisfaction and physical and mental functioning.

In summary, previous research has indicated that preparatory programmes can diminish or prevent symptoms of transfer trauma. Social support seems to be an especially important factor which can alleviate the stress associated with the move. The remainder of this chapter describes a study to investigate the possible expression of transfer trauma during the biggest single deinstitutionalization process in Finland thus far.

METHOD

The participants in this study were intellectually disabled residents of a small institution called Nastola. At the time of the institution's closure, it had 85 residents. They were of different levels on mental retardation, most subjects being profoundly handicapped. The mean age of the subjects was 35 and their average time of stay in the institution was 20 years. To analyse the results in two age groups the participants were divided in a group of 50 years or older ($N = 14$, Mean age 56, $SD = 7$) and 49 years or under ($N = 69$, $M = 33$, $SD = 9$).

The development of the adaptive behaviour of the subjects was followed using the AAMD (American Association on Mental Deficiency) Adaptive Behavior Scale (ABS) (Nihira et al., 1974). Measurements relevant to the investigation of transfer trauma were made two weeks before the closure of the institution and two weeks and six months after the residents moved into the community. Part Two of the ABS was divided into two scales according to the results of the factor analysis in a previous

Finnish study (Saloviita, 1990). The two new scales were called social and personal maladaptation, respectively. The latter scale consisted of the domains V, VI, IX, X, and XIV of Part Two.

The residents moved into small community-based group homes with five residents in each. In order to minimize the disruption of social ties during the move, the new resident groups with their own staff were already formed in the institution. The existing small living units of the institution were reorganized six months before the move according to the groupings to be used in the community.

To enhance the predictability and controllability of the move several measures were undertaken: the move was thoroughly discussed with the residents, they made visits to their new homes and participated in the furnishing and most residents participated in the farewell party.

RESULTS AND DISCUSSION

The results are presented in Tables 9.2 and 9.3. Three expressions of transfer trauma were observed: in the group with mild or moderate retardation there was an increase in personal maladaptation; in the age group of 50 years or older there was a decrease in adaptive skills; in the group with severe retardation a decrease in social maladaptation was observed. All of these effects disappeared in the follow-up studies six months later.

Using the percentage error rate formula presented by Ottenbacher (1991) it can be estimated that 30% of the statistically significant comparisons presented above were due to chance factors and the remaining 70% were likely to be a function of non-chance factors.

The occurrence of personal maladaptation among higher functioning residents is similar to results obtained by Cohen et al. (1977). The deterioration of performance with elderly people is in accordance with observations from the gerontological research. In their totality, however, the negative changes were small and lasted no longer than six months and sometimes considerably less. In addition, instant decreases in social maladaptation were observed among persons with severe retardation.

PLANNING A SMOOTH MOVE

The stressfulness of a move depends on the manner in which it is perceived by the mover and the amount of social support given. Therefore, an adequate preparatory programme should include components aimed at increasing the predictability and controllability of the move and the means with which to provide social support for the mover.

Predictability of a move can be increased in many ways. The resident

Table 0.2   The development of adaptive behaviour of persons transferred from institutions into the community by levels of mental retardation

Level of retardation Area of AB Scale	2 weeks before	2 weeks after	t	df	p
All (n=83)					
AB Part One	96.5	96.7	−0.14	82	0.892
AB Part Two	25.4	23.9	1.14	82	0.259
Social	14.7	12.9	1.75	82	0.084
Personal	10.7	11.0	−0.69	82	0.492
Mild and moderate (n=18)					
AB Part One	163.6	162.4	0.46	17	0.649
AB Part Two	22.7	25.7	−1.23	17	0.237
Social	17.4	18.1	−0.35	17	0.728
Personal	5.4	7.6	−3.03	17	0.008**
Severe (n=27)					
AB Part One	117.9	117.8	0.02	26	0.981
AB Part Two	32.2	26.3	2.28	26	0.031*
Social	21.5	16.6	2.22	26	0.035*
Personal	10.7	9.7	1.47	26	0.153
Profound (n=38)					
AB Part One	49.5	50.6	−0.67	37	0.506
AB Part Two	21.7	21.4	0.18	37	0.861
Social	8.5	7.8	0.62	37	0.538
Personal	13.2	13.7	−0.50	37	0.620

*=significant at 0.05 level

**=significant at 0.01 level

Table 9.3 The development of adaptive behaviour of persons with intellectual disabilities transferred from institutions into the community presented by age

Age group Area of AB Scale	2 weeks before	2 weeks after	t	df	p
Age 49 or under					
(n=69)					
AB Part One	88.5	90.3	−1.33	68	0.187
AB Part Two	23.7	22.9	0.67	68	0.505
Social	12.9	11.6	1.26	68	0.213
Personal	10.8	11.2	−0.75	68	0.455
Age 50 or over (n=14)					
AB Part One	135.9	128.1	2.29	13	0.039*
AB Part Two	33.4	29.3	1.09	13	0.296
Social	23.3	19.1	1.27	13	0.226
Personal	10.1	10.1	0.00	13	1.000

*=significant at 0.05 level

needs realistic information about the move, the new setting, and its conditions. Symbolic preparations can be made, for example, physical examination or purchasing of new clothes because of the move (e.g. Weinstock *et al.*, 1979). All possible problems should be thoroughly discussed with the movers. Site visits to the new place should be a normal part of the move.

Controllability of a move demands that the residents are involved in the moving process as much as possible. They should take part in the various decisions and choices concerning the moving process, help to pack their own belongings, and involve themselves in the planning and purchasing of the new furnishings.

The question of social support is critical. The transition can cause the disconnection of many important social ties. It has also been noted that institutional closures may affect negatively the morale and performance of staff. They may withdraw from their previous attachments to the residents (Heller, 1984). To minimize the social disruption it is important that the move disconnects as few social ties as possible. During the move, the resident and staff groupings should be held as intact as possible. Heller

(1984) found that those residents who moved with their chosen friends or spouses had better post-transfer adjustment. Another way to minimize social disruption is to maintain continuity in vocational and day programming (Heller, 1988). In the present study this was possible with only a small group of the residents whose move had been within the locality of their old institution.

It is noteworthy that some expressions of transfer trauma were observed in this study even though it included a comprehensive preparatory programme and a grouping policy which aimed at maximizing social support during the move. It would be premature, however, to interpret the results as indicating that preparatory programmes are not useful. On the contrary, the findings of transfer trauma in this study emphasize the continuous need to implement preparatory programmes when transfers are planned. Given the available research the priority is not to make controlled studies of transition trauma using control groups without preparatory programmes but to concentrate instead on the identification of risk factors connected with transfer trauma and the development of programmes that minimize these manifestations.

Results of deinstitutionalization in Connecticut 10

James Conroy

This is a comprehensive report of five years of research on the well-being of more than 500 people who moved from institutions to community settings in Connecticut, a state on the east coast of the United States. They were members of a group called the CARC v. Thorne Class Members.

In the late 1970s, a lawsuit was filed by the Connecticut Association for Retarded Citizens (CARC) against Governor Thorne and many other state officials and agencies. The lawsuit alleged that conditions at the state's institutional settings, particularly the Mansfield Training School, were below even the most minimal acceptable standards of quality. It further alleged that to keep people in such an institutional setting, while hundreds of other similar people were already living and thriving in community homes, would be discriminatory and unjust.

After several years of litigation, a federal magistrate approved a settlement agreement that strongly supported the plaintiffs' contentions. The settlement conceded that people should be given every opportunity to move to homes that were more integrated and more like typical family homes in regular neighbourhoods. However, the settlement also stipulated that a major longitudinal study should be mounted to track the progress and well-being of the people during and after the move.

This chapter contains the final results of that study. The entire effort can be characterized as focusing on one simple research question: Are the people who were living in large, segregated, institutions in 1985, and are now living in community-based settings, better off or worse off than they were, and in what ways and by how much?

In 1990, representatives of the Longitudinal Study visited 1335 class members at their homes, and collected quantitative data about their lives.

This chapter, however, concentrates on the 569 people who were living in large, segregated institutions in 1985, but had moved into community settings by 1990. It is important to note, however, that this number does not fully represent the overall achievement of Connecticut in changing towards a community-based residential service system. The best reflection of that is a different statistic, the percentage of people in institutions in 1985 and in 1990. In 1985, 79% of all CARC v. Thorne Class Members lived in segregated institutions, and 21% were in community settings. In 1990, only 28% of class members lived in institutions, and 72% are in the community. In reading this chapter, which is about 569 class members, it is important to keep in mind that these are not the only people whose lives have been affected by the CARC v. Thorne consent decree. The major institution involved in the case, the Mansfield Training School, is closed and all the people who once lived there have moved to new homes in the community (MacNamara, 1994).

METHODS

A battery of instruments was assembled specifically for this project. There were three packages of instruments: one for each individual, one for each home setting, and one for each family. The individual instrument package was the Connecticut Individual Evaluation Report (CIER). One was completed for each person visited. The package oriented at the setting rather than the individual was the Site Review Package. One of these packages was completed for each home visited; if several people lived at one home, only one Site Review Package was completed. Each family was offered an opportunity to complete a family survey.

This battery of instruments is based on the dual notions that 'quality of life' is inherently multidimensional (Conroy and Feinstein, 1990a), so there are many kinds of outcomes to measure, and that valued outcomes may be different for different people (Conroy and Feinstein, 1990b; Shea, 1992). Professionals may value some outcomes most highly, such as behavioural development; parents and other relatives may value permanence, safety, and comfort more highly; and people themselves may value having freedom, money, and friends most highly. The goal in this body of work and related efforts has been to learn how to measure aspects of all of these valued outcomes reliably.

Taken together, the measures in the 1990 battery included behavioural progress, integration, productivity, earnings, status of each person's written habilitation plan, health, health care, medications, amount and type of developmentally oriented services, satisfaction of the people receiving services, satisfaction of next of kin, physical quality, individualized prac-tires, staff attitudes, and programme cost. The data collection instruments, and their reliability, have been described in the Pennhurst reports and subsequent documents (Conroy and Bradley, 1985; Devlin, 1989; Lemanowicz et al., 1990; Conroy, 1994; Conroy and Seiders, 1994).

The individual package, or Connecticut Individual Evaluation Report (CIER), was developed by combining, modifying, and adding to, several other instruments already known to be reliable and valid. The behavioural items of the CIER were modified from the State of California Department of Developmental Services' Client Development Evaluation Report (1978). The California instrument covered adaptive behaviour, challenging (maladaptive) behaviour, vocational behaviour, and medical status.

The adaptive behaviour section of the CIER contained 46 items relating to: motor abilities, independent living skills, communication skills, social/emotional skills, and cognitive skills. When the item scores were summed, an adaptive behaviour sum score was produced, which was scaled to range from 0–100.

The CIER also contained 11 items on challenging behaviours, including aggression, running away, hyperactivity, etc. These 11 items were summed to produce a challenging behaviour total score. The scores were again cast in terms of a 0–100 point scale; a higher score indicated fewer challenging behaviours.

The behavioural items from the original California instrument were tested for interrater reliability by Harris (1982). In a study including 750 people in a variety of settings, the interrater reliability of the adaptive and challenging behaviour items fell almost entirely in the range from 0.70–0.95, although no average or overall score was given. For item reliabilities, such figures are well within the acceptable range. We used prior years' data (1985 and 1986) in Connecticut to examine test–retest reliability. The correlation between the 1985 and 1986 Adaptive Behavior Scale scores was 0.94; for the challenging behaviour scale it was 0.66. A third kind of reliability, internal consistency, was tested in the 1986 data, and the results were 0.97 for adaptive and 0.80 for challenging behaviour.

Items on demographics, other disabilities, family contact, medications and health, integration, productivity, services received, and consumer satisfaction, were all taken from the package that we had been using for many years in Pennsylvania.

There were two measures of integration and inclusion. The Social Presence Scale was developed specifically for the Connecticut project. It was tested in 1985 and revised in 1986. Information was collected about the frequency of opportunities for interaction between class members and non-handicapped people other than staff. It was interpretable as 'how many times per week a person got out into integrated settings'. These could include movies, grocery stores, banks, restaurants, sports events, parks, and so on. A second measure of integration was the Integrative Activities Scale. This scale was taken from the 1986 Louis Harris poll of Americans with disabilities (Taylor *et al.*, 1986). The Harris organization conducted 1000 telephone interviews with adults with disabilities, and another 1000 interviews with non-disabled members of the general population. This scale thus offered a basis for comparison and social validation. It captured how often people visited with friends or neighbours, went shopping, to a restaurant, and so on. Both of these scales really measured only half of the total dimension of integration. If integration was composed of presence in the mainstream of community life and activity, plus participation in the mainstream, then these scales only captured 'presence'. More research will be needed to produce reliable measurement approaches to integration's participation/inclusion aspects.

We included Schalock's (1989), Quality of Life Questionnaire (or QOLQ) as our individual interview. The QOLQ had been used in several other areas of the United States, and also in other countries (Schalock *et al.*, 1989). The QOLQ is designed as a direct interview of the person or whoever knows the person best. The 1990 version of the scale was composed of 40 questions arranged in four sections: Satisfaction, Competence/Productivity, Empowerment/Independence, and Social Belonging/Community Integration.

Unlike the CIER, one Site Review Package was collected for each residential setting, rather than for each person. There are certain facets of well-being that cannot be tied to any one individual, but only to the home, such as the physical quality of the home. In 1990, the package had eight sections: Size, Staff, Physical Quality, the Group Home Management Scale, Basic Life and Safety Issues, Site Reviewer Impressions, Special Concerns, and Positive Comments.

The Size section collected information about the size of the immediate environment experienced by the people who lived there. For community service providers, it also collected the size of the provider agency overall. In case the setting was a congregate care facility, the overall size of the facility was collected. These items were related to the considerable theoretical interest in the 'ideal' and most 'cost-effective' size of settings and of providers.

The Physical Quality Index (PQI) was modified from Seltzer's (1980) instrument, which was in turn a derivative of portions of the Multiphasic Environmental Rating Procedure (Moos, 1980). It was a measure of how home-like and pleasant the setting was. It was completed after the visiting data collector had walked through the residence, rating each room on dimensions such as cleanliness, odours, condition of the furniture, individualized decorations, and overall pleasantness. Interrater reliability of the PQI was reported as 0.81, with test–retest at 0.70 (Devlin, 1989).

The Group Home Management Scale (GHMS) was adapted from a scale developed by King *et al.* (1971) in England, and applied in international research by Balla (1976) and his colleagues at Yale. It was composed of only ten items, all intended to measure the degree to which the routine of life was regimented as opposed to individualized.

Site Reviewer Impressions were the purely subjective feelings of our data collectors about six dimensions of the quality of life. The six dimensions were: overall rating of the perceived overall quality of the residential site, quality of food found in the refrigerator and cupboards, quality of staff–consumer interactions, quality of consumer–consumer interactions, expectations of staff regarding individuals' potential for growth and development, and the degree to which the setting is oriented toward measurement and accountability. These ratings were give at the end of each site review, after the data collectors had met the people, learned a great deal about them and the programme, and had toured the home.

The 1986 and 1990 Family Survey forms contained 24 items. The areas covered were demographics, satisfaction with services, perceived happiness of the class member, frequency of contact, feelings about permanence, and beliefs about the person's potential for development.

RESULTS

DESCRIPTION OF THE PEOPLE WHO MOVED FROM CONGREGATE TO COMMUNITY CARE

The Longitudinal Study collected complete data about 569 class members who moved from institutions to community living situations between 1985 and 1990. For convenience in this chapter, these people will be referred to as 'movers'. Their counterparts who remained in institutional settings will be called 'stayers'.

The movers were 51% male and 49% female. Their reported ages ranged from 22–93, with a mean age of 47. Their levels of retardation broke down as 44% profound, 29% severe, 16% moderate, and 11% mild. These were clearly people who were neither young nor mildly disabled. Under this consent decree, in a 5-year period, fully 73% of community placements were people labelled severely or profoundly retarded.

The movers also experienced other disabilities. A total of 11% of them had a severe or total vision loss, 3% had a severe or total loss of hearing, and 30% used a wheelchair. In the health area, 3% 'would not survive without 24-hour medical personnel', and another 6% had 'a life-threatening condition that requires rapid access to medical care'. A history of seizures, but none currently, was reported for 17%, and another 18% have had seizures during the past year.

All in all, these descriptions demonstrated that the people who moved into the community were very seriously disabled, they were relatively old, and many of them had more than one disabling condition. These were emphatically not the kind of people who would have been described as easy to serve in the community in the past. This is an important point to keep in mind in evaluating how the quality of their lives has changed.

Table 10.1 shows the kind of facilities from which the movers came. Most of the movers came from Mansfield, but a third came from other institutions. Table 10.2 shows what kind of residential settings the movers were living in five years later, in 1990. Table 10.3 shows the kinds of daytime activities in which the movers are now engaged. One-third of the movers attended a Community Experience Program, which was geared to help them learn skills that would enhance their adaptation to, and productivity in, the community at large. One-quarter were in sheltered employment, in which they earned wages. Most remarkable was the fact that nearly one-fifth of the movers were in supported work placements, a figure that other parts of the nation would envy. In Philadelphia, for example, of the 839 people we monitored in 1990, only nine were in supported employment.

The longitudinal research design looks for changes over time. The change in adaptive behaviour is shown on the left-hand side of Figure 10.1. The 569 movers had an average adaptive behaviour score of 49.5 in 1985, when they were living in institutions. In 1990, out in their new community homes, their average score was 54.0. This gain of 4.5 points was highly statistically significant ($t=11.5$, $df=568$, $p<0.0001$) and was broadly consistent with our other research (Pennsylvania, 8% in 7 years; Louisiana, 8% in 7 years; New Hampshire, 5% in 5 years).

In the area of challenging behaviour, the average score in institutions in 1985 was 79.0, and in 1990 in the community the average score was 80.2, indicating a 1.2 point gain in the area of challenging behaviour ($t=1.5$, $df=556$, $p=0.061$, one-tailed). This small change is represented on the right-hand side of the Figure 10.1 graph. Although the change is nonsignificant it is important because we were dealing with a population and not a sample, and so inferential statistics were not strictly necessary. Therefore, any changes that were measured should be thought of as real, and our task is to interpret the practical significance of a 1.2 point change in challenging behaviour. It meant that people displayed somewhat fewer

Table 10.1 Where the movers lived in 1985

	Number of movers	%
Mansfield Training School	375	66
Regional Centre – on campus	80	14
Skilled nursing facility	67	12
Home for the aged	35	6
General intermediate care facility	9	2
Southbury Training School	3	1

Table 10.2 Type of community placements of the movers

	Number of movers	%
Group home, Non ICF/MR* (4 or more beds)	264	46
Group home, ICF/MR* (4 or more beds)	148	26
Community living arrangement (3 or fewer beds)	127	22
Supervised, supported, or co-operative, other	19	3
Community training home	11	2

* ICF/MR stands for a Federal funding programme that is part of the Social Security Act, called the Intermediate Care Facilities for [People with] Mental Retardation programme.

Table 10.3 Type of community day programmes of the movers

	Number of movers	%
Community experience programme	189	33
Sheltered employment	142	25
Support work	101	18
Senior citizen programmes	98	18
Other	22	4
Competitive employment	9	2
No day programme	6	1

challenging behaviours in the community than they did previously in institutions. Although noticeable for some people, the changes would be minor for most. Moreover, over a period of many years, such gains would add up, and would become clearly noticeable improvements.

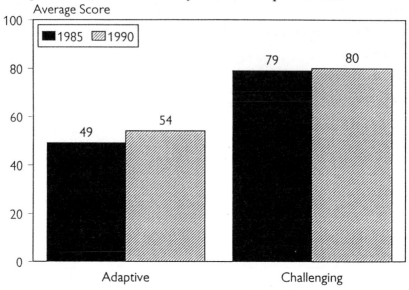

Figure 10.1 Behaviour changes among movers (longitudinal design, n=569).

Another measure of whether people are better off is health, and one indicator of general health is the use of medications. In 1985, the movers received an average of 1.6 different medications each day. In 1990, the average number of medications increased to 1.9 ($t=4.2$, $df=564$, $p<0.0001$). This increase may be a cause for concern, yet it is not dissimilar from what we have observed in other states. Many people contend that in the community people are receiving more appropriate medical care and that the medications received are needed. Others argue that medical care in the community is fragmented and lacks coordination. Hence, two physicians may often prescribe independently of one another, causing people to receive more medication than when they lived in institutions.

Another indicator of health status was this item: 'In general, how urgent is this person's need for medical care?' The responses are displayed in Table 10.4. Statistically, the changes were not significant. However, the slight increases in the 'Would not survive ... ' and 'Needs visiting nurse ... ' categories might be related to aging of the group.

Another valued outcome for all citizens, and stated explicitly in the Developmental Disabilities Assistance and Bill of Rights Act Amendments

Table 10.4 'In general, how urgent is this person's need for medical care?'

	1985 (%)	1990 (%)
Would not survive without 24-hour medical personnel	1.9	3.2
Has life-threatening condition that requires rapid access to medical care	5.3	5.7
Needs visiting nurse and/or regular doctor's visits	36.4	41.7
Has no serious medical needs	54.8	49.4

of 1987, is productivity. In the Act, productivity was defined as 'engagement in income-producing work by a person with developmental disabilities which is measured through improvements in income level, employment status, or job advancement, or, engagement by a person with developmental disabilities in work which contributes to a household or community'. The primary measure of productivity that was used throughout the Longitudinal Study was income.

Specifically, we asked how much money the individual earned in an average week. In 1985 the average among the 569 movers was $2.06; by 1990, this average had increased to $10.02 ($t=9.3$, $df=543$, $p<0.0001$). This represented almost a 500% increase over the five years. It could be argued that this 500% increase did not mean a significantly enhanced quality of life, we would argue that it did represent a significant shift in the income-producing opportunities afforded Connecticut citizens with disabilities. This shift away from segregated, non-paid opportunities, to integrated, income-producing opportunities, is illustrated in Table 10.5.

The percentage of individuals involved in supported employment increased from 1.4% in 1985 to 17.8% in 1990. In addition, the proportion of older adults involved in senior citizens' programmes jumped from 0.2% in 1985 to 17.5% in 1990 (including generic senior citizen programmes). Finally, in 1985, 18.2% of the class members (102 individuals) had no day programme/employment whatsoever. In 1990 that number dropped to 1.1% (six individuals).

A measure of the valued outcome of integration (actually of opportunities for integration rather than actual integration) was the Social Presence Scale. In 1986, in institutions, the average score was 2, and in 1990 in the community, the average score was 16 ($t=18.4$, $df=462$, $p<0.0001$). The average class member in 1990 experienced, on average, two opportunities for interaction with individuals without disabilities per day, as opposed to about two interactions per week in institutions. Insofar as integration was one of the important goals of deinstitutionalization, this finding was

Table 10.5 Employment and occupation before and after transfer

	1985 (%)	1990 (%)
Community experience	44.2	33.3
Sheltered employment	20.0	25.0
Supported work	1.4	17.8
Competitive employment	0.5	1.6
Opportunities for older adults	0.2	15.7
Generic senior citizen programmes	0.0	1.8
School programmes	5.4	0.0
Other day programmes	8.5	3.7
No day programmes	18.2	1.1

strong evidence that class members who moved to the community were much better off.

One of the other goals of deinstitutionalization was to move individuals from large, segregated settings to smaller, integrated settings in the community. The average size of the immediate living areas in institutions was 20.7 people. In the community, the average size of immediate living areas was 4.7 people ($t=28.6$, $df=565$, $p<0.0001$). Increased contact with families was another dimension that might be considered as a valued outcome. The measurement scale ranged from 1 (never) to 5 (weekly or more). The frequency of family visits to the class member increased on this scale after people moved out into the community, from an average of 2.3–2.6 ($t=5.4$, $df=361$, $p<0.0001$). On the same scale, the frequency of class member visits to the family increased from 1.8–2.0 ($t=4.4$, $df=361$, $p<0.0001$).

Another dimension was the quality of the home environments. The GHMS measured the extent to which the environment was individualized to meet the specific needs of class members, versus regimented into uniform rules for all. The GHMS was scored so that higher scores represented more individualized settings. In the institutions in 1985 the average GHMS score was 5.3, and in the community in 1990 the average score was 16.5 ($t=36.84$, $df=391$, $p<0.0001$). In other words, the movers were experiencing much more individualized treatment in their homes in the community than they had at the institutions.

The Physical Quality Instrument average score in 1985 in institutions was 60.6, and in 1990 in the community the average score was 67.8 ($t=11.4$, $df=532$, $p<0.0001$). The average community setting was rated as considerably higher in physical quality than the average institutional setting.

Table 10.6 Site reviewer ratings

	1985	1990
Overall, how would you rate this site? (1=poor, 10=excellent)	5.4	7.9*
How would you rate the quality and quantity of food in the refrigerator and cupboards? (1=poor, 10=excellent)	5.8	8.2*
How to you perceive staff–consumer/consumer–staff interactions? (1=cold, impersonal, 10=warm, personal)	7.2	8.3*
How do you perceive consumer–consumer interactions? (1−unfriendly, 10−friendly)	5.0	6.8*
What are staff's expectations for consumers regarding growth? (1=pessimistic, 10=enthusiastic)	5.5	7.8*
To what extent is this setting oriented toward measurement, research and scientific approaches? (1=not at all, 10=as much as I've ever seen)	4.1	6.4*

* = significant at <0.0001

The Site Reviewer Impressions, although subjective, were intended to capture the personal impressions of the experienced visitors. The results are displayed in Table 10.6 and show that site reviewers believed that the community settings were considerably better than the institutions from which people came.

MATCHED COMPARISON RESULTS

The longitudinal design enabled us to learn that the movers were better off in the community than they were in 1985 in most of the measured areas. But perhaps the stayers were also better off, because the institutions had also improved during the five years. To check for this possibility, we needed to compare the changes experienced by the movers and the stayers. Since the movers and stayers differed (stayers had significantly lower adaptive behaviour, more challenging behaviour and more urgent need for medical care) a matched comparison study was undertaken to examine this question.

We attempted to find a match for each of the 340 stayers in the pool of 569 movers. The characteristics matched were adaptive behaviour, challenging behaviour, medical needs, and age. For each stayer, we tried to find a mover with adaptive behaviour within ten points; challenging behaviour within five points; age within ten years; and the same degree of medical needs. We were able to find exact matches for 124 of the stayers, using these criteria. T-tests revealed no significant differences between the groups of movers and stayers in 1985 on any of the four matching variables.

By 1990, the two groups were significantly different on several variables. In adaptive behaviour the movers averaged 47 in adaptive behaviour and the stayers averaged 41 ($t=2.09$, $df=242$, $p=0.038$). On the Social Presence Scale, the movers averaged 13 and the stayers 5 ($t=5.26$, $df=246$, $p<0.0001$). On the Harris Poll Scale, the movers scored 35 and the stayers scored 17 ($t=9.98$, $df=239$, $p<0.0001$). On the Quality of Life Questionnaire total scale scores, the movers averaged 76, and the stayers 69 ($t=4.42$, $df=172$, $p<0.0001$).

There were three questions about staff attitudes to compare. In the first question, on a 1–10 scale, staff were asked to rate: 'How much do you like this job?' The community-based staff of the movers averaged 9.1, and the institutions' staff of the stayers averaged 8.6, on this subjective rating ($t=3.03$, $df=239$, $p=0.003$). In a related item, staff were asked to rate: 'How much do you like working with this person?' on the same 1–10 scale. Again, the ratings were high, with the movers' staff scoring 8.9 and stayers' staff 8.1, but the differences were still significant ($t=4.17$, $df=243$, $p<0.0001$). Another item rated by staff was a scale which addressed 'the progress made by this person in the past year'. A '1' meant they regressed a lot, and '10' meant they progressed a lot. The movers' staff persons rated an average of 8.6 on this item, compared to 7.4 for the stayers' staff ($t=5.06$, $df=244$, $p<0.0001$).

Moving to environmental quality indicators, we compared the size of the immediate residential setting for movers and stayers. On the average, stayers were living in immediate proximity to 11 people; for movers, the figure was 4 ($t=16.74$, $df=246$, $p<0.001$). On the Group Home Management Survey, the community settings averaged 14, and the institutions averaged 10 ($t=5.49$, $df=182$, $p<0.0001$). The average Physical Quality Index score for movers was 68, compared to 54 for the stayers ($t=12.17$, $df=231$, $p<0.0001$). Finally, the subjective opinions of data collectors were examined. There were six ratings, all on ten point scales. The results are shown in Figure 10.2. Ratings assigned to the movers were higher on all six items, and every difference was significant beyond the 0.005 level.

There were some indicators of quality and services that showed no significant differences between movers and stayers: these were challenging behaviour, number of weeks since the case manager visited, number of medications taken daily, level of need for medical care, hours per week attending the day programme, frequency of visits from or to family members and earnings per week.

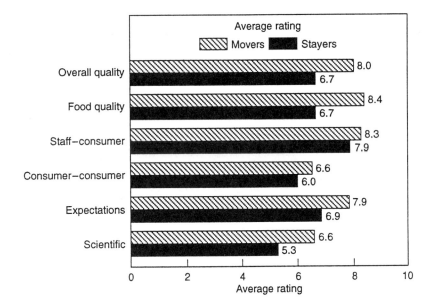

Figure 10.2 Six subjective ratings of quality (matched comparison, 124 pairs).

The health indicators were interesting in that the longitudinal analysis appeared to show a trend toward increasing need for medical care over time, which might indicate declining health. In the matched comparison design, however, statistical tests showed that movers and stayers were equally in need of health care in 1985 and again in 1990. Similarly, we were unable to confirm a statistically significant change over time on this variable, for either the movers or the stayers. We therefore conclude that the matched comparison does not confirm the evidence of declining health seen in the longitudinal analysis. We also conclude that there have been no changes in medical needs over time, for either group. Similarly, the matched comparison analysis failed to detect a difference in the number of medications being given daily to movers and stayers, and thus did not confirm the longitudinal finding of increased medications among the movers.

More information about the content of services is provided by Figure 10.3. This shows the service delivery pattern as prescribed in the Overall Plan of Services (OPS). For each of 17 services, information was recorded about whether the service was in the OPS, whether the service was delivered and whether the amount was sufficient. Information was only collected for those services that were formally structured and scheduled.

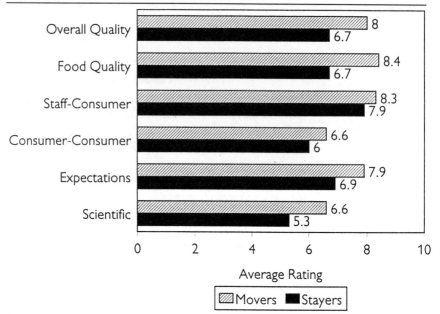

Figure 10.3 Number of people receiving each service (matched comparison, 124 pairs).

Stayers were slightly more likely to have medical/nursing services specified in the OPS, but overall, medical/nursing was in almost everyone's written plan. In the community, hygiene skills training was the second most common, and it was much more common than in the institutions. Appropriate social behaviour training and communication skills training were the next most frequently prescribed in both types of setting. Community living and domestic skills training, however, were far more prevalent among the movers. Recreation skills training (defined as a service designed by a recreation therapist but delivered by a direct care staff person) was far more common among stayers. Correspondingly, the services of a recreation therapist were more likely to be received by stayers. Apparently, there was significant emphasis in the recreation area in Connecticut's institutional settings.

Eating and mobility service patterns were similar for movers and stayers. Movers tended to get more training in sensorimotor skills and dressing skills. Speech therapy and physical therapy were about equally common for movers and stayers. Occupational therapy and counselling/psychotherapy, although not very common services, were more common in the community than in institutions. Finally, cognitive skills training was more often received by stayers than movers.

FAMILY SURVEY RESULTS

When the CIER instruments were collected in 1990 during the site visits, we also collected the name and address of the parents, close relatives, or guardians of each class member. We were able to obtain 1157 addresses for the 1335 class members. The remainder of class members either had no close family or the family did not desire contact. When the survey was complete, we had obtained 424 valid survey forms. In addition, 226 packages were returned to us because of inaccurate or outdated addresses. This translated into a response rate of 46%, which was typical of single-round mail surveys of this type (Conroy, 1992).

There were 255 families who responded to the survey both in 1986 and 1990. Of those 255, 101 had relatives who were in institutions in 1986, but had moved to community settings by 1990. Respondents were the mother in 28 cases, a sibling in 24 cases, the mother and father together in 23 cases, the father in 12 cases, a guardian in 8 cases and others in the remaining 6 cases. The items on the family survey fell into four groups of issues: satisfaction and quality, security and permanence, visits, and attitudes about individual development.

Figure 10.4 summarizes the changes in nine items related to satisfaction and quality of life from 1986–1990. All of these changes were statistically significant (by paired t-tests, using the 0.05 level of significance criterion). For items that were worded negatively, we reversed the scoring system so that higher numbers were always favourable on the graph. Families were very highly satisfied with their relatives' institutions in 1986. However, they reported even higher satisfaction with community services in 1990. The fact that every item increased significantly demonstrated that the effect was very strong and uniform.

Figure 10.5 shows which of the families' perceptions appeared to have changed the most since community placement. The perception that the class member had adequate privacy was the greatest change, with satisfaction with the residence coming in second.

Because it is well recognized that security and permanence are at or near the top of the list of families' concerns about their relatives' lives (Latib et al., 1984), the family survey included three items concerning permanence. There was no significant change in any of these three items from 1986 institutions to 1990 community living. On the funding item, families on average were 'in between' agreement and disagreement that funding was secure and permanent. Actually, this was an interesting finding. One might have expected higher confidence in the 'bricks and mortar' of the old 'tried and true' institutions than in the new community home models. This was not the case. Confidence in funding was just

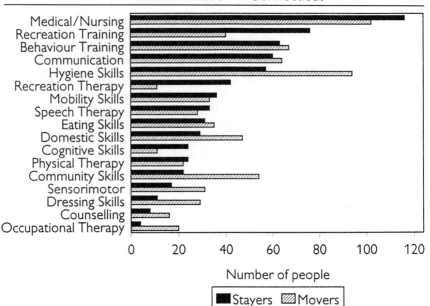

Figure 10.4 Survey of movers' families: perceived changes 1986–90 (n=101).

about the same when people moved out into the community. The question about whether the relatives' service provider would still be in business five years in the future also did not change. Again, one might have expected a decrease in confidence on this item. Training Schools and Regional Centres might have been perceived as more stable than group homes. This did not turn out to be true. On average, families tended to feel weak agreement with the five years' statement. Finally, families did not change in their initially very strong concern that: 'It is very important that I have the major say about what happens to my relative'. This concern was initially strong, and it remained strong even after community placement. The mean score on the five point scale was 4.13 in 1986, and 4.27 in 1990.

To summarize the family survey findings, families were more satisfied with community residential and day settings than they were with the previous institutions. They also believed their relatives were happier with both residential and day programmes. Families of community movers were more trusting of staff, less concerned about turnover, less concerned that they were not getting the medical care they need, they believed their relatives were getting better food, they believed their relatives had more privacy in their community homes, and they had just as much confidence in the permanence of the community homes as they previously did in the

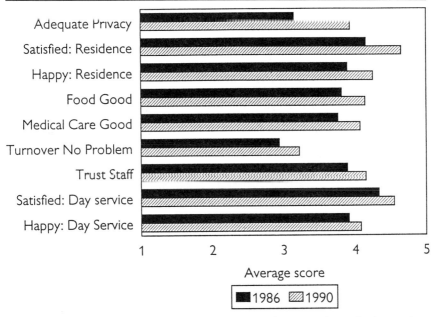

Figure 10.5 Survey of movers' families: magnitude of changes in quality (n=101).

institutional settings. They continued to want to have a strong and respected voice in determining what happened to their loved ones.

CONCLUSION

The Longitudinal Study of the CARC v. Thorne Class Members was responsible for visiting 1298 class members in 1985, 1342 in 1986, 1344 in 1987, 1335 in 1989, and 1335 in 1990. This chapter has focused on people who were visited in 1985, and were living in institutions, and who then moved to community settings, and were visited again in 1990. We applied three major research designs (longitudinal, matched comparison, and family survey), all aimed at the question of whether people were 'better off'. But two of the designs approached the question in slightly different ways. The longitudinal design asked whether people who moved into the community were better off in 1990 than they had been in 1985. The matched comparison design asked whether people who moved into the community were better off in 1990 than very similar people who were still in institutions.

The results of the entire study have been summarized in Table 10.7. Since both designs yield similar findings, we can be very confident in the validity of the results. The overwhelming picture is positive.

Table 10.7 Consumer outcomes associated with deinstitutionalization, Connecticut, 1985–91

	Matched comparison design	Longitudinal design	Family survey
Adaptive behaviour improvement	++	++	
Challenging behaviour improvement	0	+	
Intensity of medical needs	0	–	
Reduced daily medications	0	–	
Increased earnings	0	+	
Day programme productivity	+	++	
Subjective quality ratings	++	++	
Individualized treatment	++	++	
Physical quality of residence	++	+	
Social presence (integration)	++	++	
Harris integration scale	++		
Quality of life questionnaire	++		
Frequency of case manager visits	0	+	
Staff like their jobs	+		
Staff like working with person	+		
Staff think person has progressed	+		
Family visits to person	0	+	0
Person visits with family	0	+	0
Family satisfaction, residence			++
Family satisfaction, day programme			+
Family perception, happiness, home			++
Family perception, happiness, day			+
Family trust in staff competence			+

++ Extremely positive finding
+ Positive finding
0 Neutral finding
– Negative finding
– Extremely negative finding

There were only two negative findings to be reported. One negative aspect was that the number of daily medications increased slightly from 1985–1990 in the longitudinal design. The 569 people we tracked during their move from institution to community were receiving a higher number of daily medications in the community than they did in 1985 in institutions. However, this finding seemed to be a general pattern for all class members, both movers and stayers. The matched comparison analysis showed that there was no difference between movers and stayers in the number of daily medications taken in 1990; the number of daily medications increased for both movers and stayers between 1985 and 1990. This suggested that the effect may have been a simple function of aging.

The only other negative finding was the increased urgency of medical needs between 1985 and 1990 in the longitudinal design. For the 569 movers, the reported intensity of medical care needed was slightly greater in 1990 than it was in 1985 in institutions. Again, the matched comparison design revealed no difference between movers and stayers in 1990. The urgency of medical needs seemed to have increased for both movers and stayers, although for neither group was the change statistically significant.

In every other dimension we measured, people were either no worse off or considerably better off in 1990 than they were in 1985. In both the matched comparison and longitudinal designs, people were better off in terms of adaptive behaviour than they were in 1985. This finding mirrored those from other states with a small variation in the magnitude of change. In neither the matched comparison nor the longitudinal design was there any significant change in challenging behaviour.

One of the most significant areas of improvement over the five years in Connecticut was the area of productivity and vocational activity. On almost every element measured within the employment/day programme domain, positive results were seen. People were experiencing more valued employment/day programme experiences, were earning more money (both movers and stayers), and had more opportunities for integration with non-handicapped people during day programmes/employment.

Integration was affected dramatically by deinstitutionalization. Both the longitudinal and the matched comparison design showed sharp increases in our measures of social presence and social integration. The members of the class were much more integrated after moving from institutions to community settings.

On Schalock's Quality of Life Questionnaire, the matched comparison revealed that movers consistently gave higher ratings than matched stayers. To the degree that this scale was reflective of the elusive concept of quality of life, people who moved to the community were better off.

Case management evidently evolved considerably during the course of this study. The longitudinal design revealed that case managers were visiting more often than they used to. The matched comparison design showed that this was true for both movers and matched stayers; case managers were visiting more often than before, both in congregate and community settings.

The matched comparison design included new questions for staff about how they like their job, how they like working with the specific class member, and whether they have seen progress in the class member. All three results favoured the movers over the stayers.

The second group of outcomes were related more to the residential environments than to individuals. Both research designs showed strong superiority of the community settings on all measures. We conclude that class members in the community were better off than they were before, and better off than similar people who were still awaiting community placement. We also infer that community residential settings were clearly 'better' than institutions in all the environmental dimensions we measured.

With regard to the frequency of family contact, often thought to be a valued outcome of returning to the community, our findings were mixed. Certainly family visits have not decreased. The matched comparison design showed that matched movers and stayers had about the same level of contact with their families.

The family survey showed that family satisfaction with the relative's new home in the community was significantly greater than their previous satisfaction with institution living units. It should be emphasized that prior satisfaction with the institutions was high, and that about half of the families in our analysis initially opposed community placement for their relatives. Once their relatives were out in the community, the satisfaction of the families was even higher than it was before. Satisfaction with their relative's day programme was also greater in 1990 than it was in 1986 in institutions. On every measure related to quality on the family survey, ratings improved significantly for the people who moved to the community. Clearly, the families of the movers believed strongly that these members of the CARC v. Thorne class were better off living in the community.

In summary, the evidence from five years of study, using three different research approaches, was very clear and consistent. The answer to the question posed at the beginning of this chapter is that the people who moved from institutions to community settings were, on average, much better off in almost every way we measured. We conclude that the opportunity to live and work in regular communities, and to construct regular lives, should be offered to every class member as soon as possible.

Impact of deinstitution-alization on service users in Britain

11

Eric Emerson and Chris Hatton

Between 1980 and 1991 the numbers of people with learning disabilities living in state-operated mental handicap hospitals in Britain fell from approximately 56 000 to 30 000. Approximately 70% of the remaining hospitals in England are currently scheduled for closure by the year 2000 which, when combined with the planned contraction of remaining institutions, should result in a further 67% reduction of provision in hospital-based residential provision by the end of the century (Greig, 1993; Chapter 1).

These broad statistics do, however, mask some important variation. The pace and nature of deinstitutionalization has varied widely between and within countries in Britain (Hunter and Wistow, 1987). In general, the replacement of large-scale institutional provision began earlier and has proceeded on a more widespread basis in England than in Wales, Scotland or Northern Ireland. Thus, over the period 1980–91 percentage decline in institutional populations for the four home countries was 51% for England, 24% for Scotland, 41% for Wales and 32% for Northern Ireland.

Secondly, the nature of the services developed to replace institutional provision has varied over time and across locations. In very general terms, the first wave of deinstitutionalization in Britain involved the move of those individuals with the least severe disabilities to a range of settings including pre-existing community-based hostels, semi-supported group living, family placement schemes and independent living arrangements (cf. Korman and Glennerster, 1990; Malin, 1987). Over the last two decades attention has switched to the development of alternative forms of residential provision for people with more severe learning disabilities, including those with additional needs such as sensory impairments or challenging behaviour. This latter phase of the deinstitutionalization movement has been accompanied by considerable (and often acrimonious) debate concerning the appropriateness of different forms of residential provision for the most severely disabled (Blunden and Allen, 1987; Department of Health and Social Security, 1984; Department of Health, 1989a; 1993).

In general, initial experiments with purpose built 20–24 place residential units (e.g. Felce *et al.*, 1980) have given way in most areas to a reliance on the provision of staff support within 'ordinary' domestic scale housing for groups of 2–8 people (e.g. Felce, 1989; Lowe and de Paiva, 1991). The vast majority of these services are based upon a notion of providing a 'home for life' in which changes in the support needs of individual users can be effectively managed, rather than as a component of a developmental or transitional 'continuum' of services.

Accounting for such changes in policy in Britain towards residential provision for people with learning disabilities is problematic. Competing (though not necessarily mutually exclusive) explanations have focused on the roles played by general and specific political, social, ideological, professional and economic factors (e.g. Korman and Glennerster, 1990; Martin, 1984; Scull, 1977). Of particular interest within Britain has been the extent to which these changes, or at least the rhetoric surrounding them, have been influenced by the concepts of normalization and social role valorization (Emerson, 1992; Nirje, 1992; Wolfensberger, 1992), particularly as elaborated by O'Brien (e.g. O'Brien and Tyne, 1981) and in an influential series of working parties organized by the King's Fund (Blunden and Allen, 1987; King's Fund, 1980; 1984; 1989). Indeed, many of the notions underlying these concepts have come to be reflected in statements of local, regional and national policy (e.g. Department of Health, 1989b; Guy's Health District, 1981; North Western Regional Health Authority, 1983).

It is our intention in this chapter to provide an overview of the results of British research concerning the effects of these policy changes on the life experiences of people with learning disabilities. The importance of occasionally standing back and 'taking stock' of the impact of changes in policy is, in many ways, self-evident. It appears in this instance to be particularly important on three counts. Firstly, as noted above, there exists no clear consensus regarding the forces driving the deinstitutionalization movement. Do the changes described above simply reflect minor adjustments or accommodations in the processes by which society exerts control over a deviant group? Alternatively, are we witnessing a significant humanization of the ways in which society cares for some of its most vulnerable members? Examining the actual impact of recent changes in policy may help frame a partial answer to such questions.

Secondly, the deinstitutionalization movement itself has been characterized by intense debate concerning the most appropriate forms of residential provision for people with the most severe disabilities. In this process professionals, managers and researchers have made extensive personal investment in advocating for particular models of care. Indeed, for some, reputations and careers are based upon the purported success of the deinstitutionalization movement in general or on the presumed superiority of particular approaches to the design of community-based alternatives. An obvious danger exists that those who have been closely involved in this process will come to accept the rhetoric, rather than investigate the reality, of the policy options in question.

Finally, a number of factors coincide to make reviewing the outcomes of the deinstitutionalization movement in Britain particularly timely. The organization of health and welfare services in Britain is undergoing a period of rapid and far-reaching change resulting from the enactment of the 1990 NHS (National Health Service) and Community Care Act and the disbandment of key administrative tiers within the NHS. There is a real risk that the subsequent reallocation of roles and responsibilities may result in a loss of leadership and expertise, especially in those agencies responsible for commissioning services and strategic planning. In addition, the early identification of the deinstitutionalization movement with institutional closure has encouraged a belief among some senior managers and policy makers that, as this specific task is nearing completion, attention (and resources) may usefully be diverted to competing priorities on the social agenda, including, for example, growing media and public opposition to the closure of psychiatric hospitals in Britain.

THE STUDIES REVIEWED

The review covered research studies which evaluated the effects of deinstitutionalization in Britain and were published during the period 1980–93. Potential studies were identified through on-line searches of the Social Sciences Citation Index and PsycLit, inspection of references cited in published reports and discussion with active researchers in Britain. Studies were included if they provided quantitative or qualitative data on aspects of user-related outcomes in either hospital or community-based residential or day care, or involved evaluations of the deinstitutionalization process.

This process identified 70 publications from over 45 separate studies which examined some aspect of the effect of deinstitutionalization on the lives of approximately 2250 people with learning disabilities. A breakdown by year of publication and type of service evaluated is provided below in Figure 11.1. As can be seen, while the nature of replacement services involved in the deinstitutionalization process has varied, the majority of (in particular recent) studies have focused on comparisons of hospital-based institutional care and community-based staffed housing.

A breakdown of the degree of disability, age and gender of service users participating in these studies, where specified, is provided in Table 11.1.

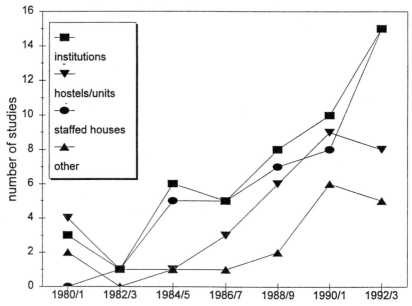

Figure 11.1 Types of services evaluated by year of publication.

Table 11.1 Age, gender and level of disability of participants (%)

Gender	Men	59
	Women	41
Age	Children	6
	Adults	73
	Unspecified	21
Level of disability	Mild/moderate	13
	Severe/profound	34
	Mixed	31
	Unspecified	21

Measures of outcome used in the studies were categorized according to a number of general domains (Figure 11.2). These were selected on the basis of O'Brien's notion of key service accomplishments (O'Brien, 1987) and broader conceptualizations of the notion of quality of life (cf. Emerson, 1985; Parmenter, 1992; Schalock, 1990).

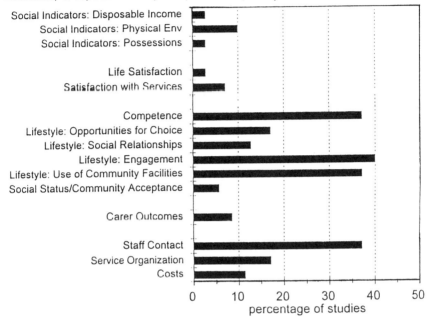

Figure 11.2 Outcomes and processes evaluated in British research on deinstitutionalization 1980–93.

These domains included:

- general social indicators of the user's quality of life with regard to disposable income (e.g. Walker *et al.*, 1993), aspects of the physical environment provided by services (e.g. Felce *et al.*, 1985) and the numbers and types of personal possessions held by service users (e.g. Davies, 1988);
- user's expressed satisfaction with regard to the services provided (e.g. Knapp *et al.*, 1992) and their overall quality of life (e.g. Stanley and Roy, 1988);
- the competence of service users (e.g. Lowe and de Paiva, 1991);
- opportunities for choice available to service users (e.g. Cattermole *et al.*, 1988);
- social relationships of service users (e.g. Malin, 1982);
- the participation of service users in community-based activities (e.g. de Kock *et al.*, 1988);

- the social status or acceptance by the community of service users (e.g. McConkey *et al.*, 1993);
- the engagement or participation of service users in everyday activities (e.g. Felce *et al.*, 1980; 1986).

In addition, six studies (8.6% of the total) assessed secondary outcomes relating to such issues as the satisfaction or stress experienced by staff or informal carers (e.g. Emerson, Cooper, Hatton *et al.*, 1993). A number of studies also included formal measures of service processes such as the quantity and nature of staff support provided to users (e.g. Orlowska *et al.*, 1991), aspects of service organization (e.g. Hewson and Walker, 1992) and service costs (e.g. Shiell *et al.*, 1992).

The review examined in greater detail those studies which examined the effects of moving from:

- large institution to medium sized community units or specialized hospital-based units (20 studies involving approximately 650 service users);
- large institution to small-scale staffed housing services (34 studies; approximately 1200 users);
- medium sized community units to small-scale staffed housing services (9 studies; 100 users).

For each study, the results pertaining to each outcome measure utilized were categorized as reflecting a significant improvement, no change, or a significant deterioration on the move from the more institutional to the less institutional setting. This categorization was based on either the report of a statistically significant difference between service models or, for three purely qualitative studies, the presence of an unqualified and unambiguous statement concerning differences between service models.

In the following sections we will summarize the results of this analysis for the most frequently used outcome domains.

THE IMPACT OF DEINSTITUTIONALIZATION

ENGAGEMENT

Direct observation of the extent of user engagement or participation in everyday activities has been the most frequent user-related outcome measure employed in British research over the past 14 years (e.g. Bratt and Johnston, 1988; Emerson *et al.*, 1992, 1993; Felce *et al.*, 1980; 1986; Hemming, Lavender and Pill, 1981; Mansell, 1994; Mansell and Beasley,

1990; Rawlings, 1985). The definition of engagement has been used with sufficient consistency in Britain to allow for the comparison of results across, as well as within, studies. Figure 11.3 presents such a comparison for all studies from which data relating to overall levels of engagement was available. Each bar represents data pertaining to either the study as a whole or, where available, data pertaining to each distinct residential unit evaluated. Figure 11.4 presents the average levels of engagement (weighted for numbers of participants per study) observed in each type of service model. It should be noted that the data in Figures 11.3 and 11.4 are based on studies rather than publications. This is of some importance given the occasional occurrence of repeated presentations of the same data across multiple publications.

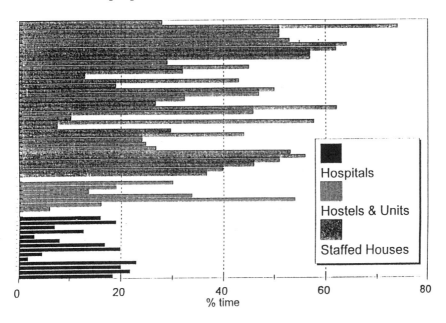

Figure 11.3 Percentage of time service users are engaged in ongoing activities across studies and service models.

As can be seen, while overall levels of engagement were higher in community-based staffed houses (weighted mean: 47.7%) than either community-based hostels and hospital-based units (24.7%) or NHS mental handicap hospitals (13.7%) significant variation occurred within each type of service. Thus, for example, the range of engagement data for each service model was 2%–23% for hospitals, 6%–54% for hostels/units and 8%–74% for community-based staffed houses. A one-way analysis of vari-

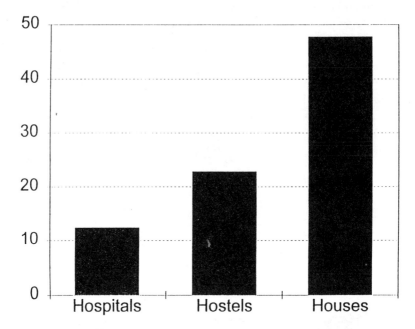

Figure 11.4 Weighted mean percentage of time service users are engaged in ongoing activities across service models.

ance of engagement by setting (hospital, hostel/unit, staffed house) revealed significant differences in levels of engagement between settings (f=18.85, df=55, p<0.0001), with *post hoc* Scheffe Tests showing that levels of engagement in staffed houses were significantly higher than levels of engagement in hostels/units and hospitals, which did not differ significantly from each other.

The frequent failure of studies to present adequate descriptive data concerning potentially significant facility and user characteristics combines with the relatively small number of studies to preclude the use of statistical procedures to identify variables which may account for the observed variation. However, Felce (Chapter 8) has reported that up to 82% of the variation in engagement data across individuals within a number of studies may be accounted for by two factors: the competence of service users and the amount of assistance (instructions, guidance, prompting) received from staff. Re-analysis of the data presented in Emerson, Cooper, Hatton *et al.* (1993) similarly indicates that up to 52% of within-participant variation in engagement data may be accounted for by the rate of assistance received by staff. Anecdotal evidence tends to suggest that those services in which high levels of staff assistance are provided are characterised

not by the presence of additional staff resources, but by the implementation of a behaviourally-orientated model of providing 'whole-environment' or 'active' support (Felce, 1988, 1991; Mansell 1995).

It is unlikely, however, that differences in the competencies of users
can account alone for the reported differences between types of service
provision as similar patterns of results are obtained from both longitudinal and comparison-group based studies. Figure 11.5 presents a summary
of within-study differences for those 15 longitudinal or 11 comparison

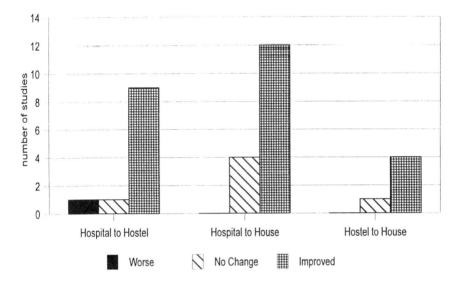

Figure 11.5 Change in user engagement in ongoing activities across service
models.

group studies which have directly compared levels of engagement in two
or more types of services.

While most comparisons (79%) made within these studies reported significantly increased levels of engagement in 'less restrictive' environments, a minority of studies, including 27% of comparisons between
hospitals and community-based staffed housing reported no significant
change. (These and all subsequent figures are based on the number of
comparisons made within studies which, due to some studies involving
comparisons between more than two types of service model, may be
greater than the number of studies quoted.)

PRESENCE AND PARTICIPATION

Twenty studies included comparisons across types of service models of user levels of participation in community-based activities. Most commonly, such studies assessed the use of community-based facilities (e.g. banks, shops, cinemas) either retrospectively (e.g. Dockrell *et al.*, 1993) or prospectively using some form of carer-completed diary (e.g., Fleming and Stenfert Kroese, 1990). While variations in procedures do not allow

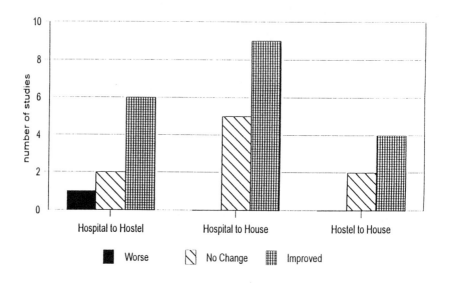

Figure 11.6 Change in user participation in community-based activities across service models.

for valid comparisons between studies, within-study comparisons reveal a pattern of results similar to those reported above (Figure 11.6).

Thus, while the majority of comparisons (66%) reported a significantly increased use of community-based facilities in less restrictive environments, a minority of studies (31%), including 36% of comparisons between hospitals and community-based staffed housing reported no change. One study (Hemming, Lavender and Pill, 1981) reported significantly less use of community-based facilities in staffed houses on a hospital site when compared with mental handicap hospital wards.

PERSONAL GROWTH

Twenty-four studies examined aspects of the personal competence of service users, primarily through the use of carer-completed questionnaires and rating scales (e.g. Fleming and Stenfert Kroese, 1990). Of these, 21

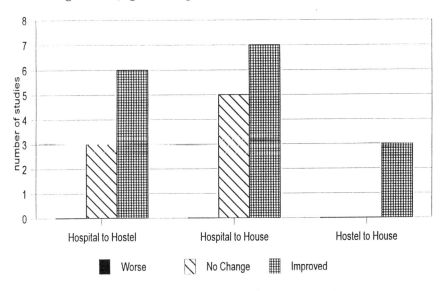

number of studies

Hospital to Hostel   Hospital to House   Hostel to House

■ Worse   ◹ No Change   ▦ Improved

Figure 11.7 Change in user competence (adaptive behaviours) across service models.

studies included 24 separate comparisons of user competence across different types of service models (e.g. Felce *et al.*, 1986).

As can be seen in Figure 11.7, while increased developmental gains were associated with purportedly less restrictive environments, for a significant minority (33%) of comparisons (including 42% of comparisons between hospitals and staffed houses) no statistically significant differences were apparent between different models of care.

OVERCOMING CHALLENGING BEHAVIOURS

Two complementary approaches have been taken to evaluating the relationship between models of service provision and changes in the extent and nature of challenging behaviours shown by service users. The majority of studies (involving 14 comparisons) evaluated change in challenging behaviour through information solicited from key informants (e.g. Murphy and Clare, 1991). A minority of studies (involving 11 separate comparisons) employed direct observational methods to measure changes in the amount of time users exhibited challenging behaviours (e.g. Emerson, Cooper, Hatton *et al.*, 1993). The results of these approaches are summarized in Figures 11.8 and 11.9.

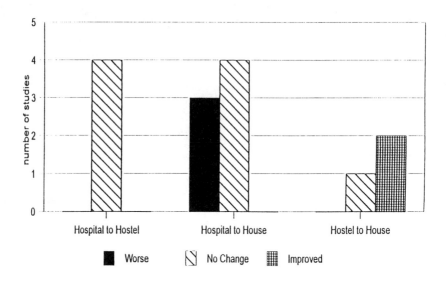

Figure 11.8 Change in reported levels of user challenging behaviours across service models.

As can be seen, the method used to assess challenging behaviour would appear to exert a strong influence over the results obtained. In general, use of key informant interviews tended to reveal a pattern of no change (64% of comparisons), although a significant minority (43%) of comparisons between hospitals and staffed housing noted a significant increase in challenging behaviours on move to smaller community-based services. In contrast, those studies which employed observational methods report an overall pattern of reduced challenging behaviour in community-based services, although this was only the case for 43% of comparisons between hospital-based provision and small community-based staffed housing.

A number of factors may account for these discrepancies. Firstly, reprovision of hospital-based care in small-scale domestic housing projects has most commonly involved the appointment and training of new staff groups rather than the transfer of both staff and users. As such, any changes in staff reports across settings may reflect either changes in the behaviour of users or the attitudes and expectations of informants towards deviant behaviour. This may be particularly significant given the use of 'values-based' training to raise the expectations of, primarily inexperienced and unqualified, support staff in community-based-services (cf. Towell, 1988; Towell and Beardshaw, 1991).

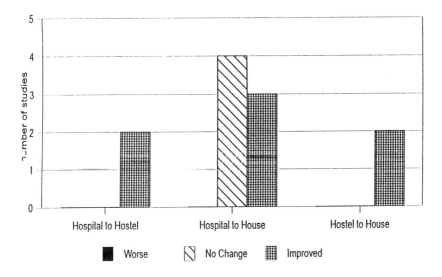

Figure 11.9 Change in observed levels of user challenging behaviours across service models.

Secondly, discrepancy between methods may reflect differing patterns of change among different types of challenging behaviour. Thus, for example, observational measures based on estimating the duration of behaviour may be particularly sensitive to changes in stereotypic behaviours which may be expected to reduce in more enriched environments (cf. Horner, 1980). Interview-based approaches, however, are likely to sample a wider range of behaviours, including low frequency short duration but high intensity behaviours which staff may well find challenging. There is little evidence, of course, to suggest that the occurrence of more seriously challenging behaviours is systematically associated with general levels of environmental stimulation. Indeed, there exists accumulating evidence that, while the motivational bases underlying seriously challenging behaviours are undoubtedly complex and diverse (Murphy, 1993), such factors as social avoidance or escape from carer-mediated demands may underlie many examples of severe self-injurious and aggressive behaviours (e.g. Derby *et al.*, 1992; Emerson, 1990).

CONCLUSIONS

In general, it is apparent that the move from institutions to smaller, community-based services has been associated with gains in the areas of user engagement in everyday activities, participation in community-based activities, personal growth and reductions in observed (probably stereo-typic) challenging behaviour. It is also apparent, however, that these are far from inevitable consequences of deinstitutionalization and that significant variation exists in the quality of community-based provision. Indeed, for a significant minority of studies (and hence individuals) life in the community would appear to be relatively indistinguishable, on these measures of outcome at least, from life in institutional provision.

While such observations are of clear importance, this overview of the available evidence is in many ways more illuminating for the questions it leaves unanswered. These include questions pertaining to the determinants of quality in community-based services, the longer-term impact of deinstitutionalization and normative judgements concerning the adequacy or acceptability of alternatives to institutional provision.

DETERMINANTS OF QUALITY

The vast majority of research on the effects of deinstitutionalization in Britain has involved small-scale comparisons between two, or occasionally three, types of service model. This, when combined with the lack of comparability of measures across studies, takes the identification of determinants of quality in replacement services into the realms of speculation. Nevertheless, three factors may be identified as being of potential significance.

Firstly, the human and financial resources available within the setting are likely to be related to overall service quality. It is readily apparent, however, that no simple relationship exists between resources and quality. Thus, for example, although some studies have reported a weak overall association between the quality and costs of residential services (e.g. Cambridge *et al.*, 1994; Shiell *et al.*, 1993), other studies have either failed to find any such overall association (e.g. Emerson, Cooper, Hatton *et al.*, 1993) or have failed to identify any significant improvements in quality associated with the addition of significant resources (e.g. Emerson *et al.*, 1992). This latter observation is, of course, consistent with the extensive literature pointing to the tenuous relationship between staffing ratios and staff:client interaction (e.g. Felce *et al.*, 1991; Seys and Duker, 1988) and the frequent failure of enhancing human resources through staff training to influence actual staff performance (e.g. Reid *et al.*, 1989). It would appear that an adequate level of resources may be a necessary but certainly not sufficient condition for providing high quality residential care.

This suggests that internal organizational structures to ensure the efficient and appropriate utilization of resources are likely to play a particularly significant role in determining the actual quality of care provided within a setting. Thus, for example, Felce (1988; 1991; Chapter 8) and others (Mansell, Chapter 4; McGill and Toogood, 1993) have argued that the implementation of an 'active support' model through clearly defined structures for planning staff and user activity are an essential component of high quality residential provision. It is also clear, however, that the adoption of such a model is often (although possibly mistakenly) seen as being in conflict with the implementation of the concepts of normalization and social role valorization (Emerson and McGill, 1989; McGill and Emerson, 1992).

Finally, key leadership is likely to be of considerable importance in acquiring and sustaining sufficient resources, establishing appropriate internal structures and motivating staff to implement the procedures necessary to ensure quality lifestyles for people with learning disabilities (Mansell, Chapter 4). The importance of effective leadership in key roles is suggested by evidence highlighting service decay over time (e.g. Blunden and Evans, 1988; Woods and Cullen, 1983) and the apparent reduction in quality associated with the more widespread implementation of the staffed housing model (Mansell, Chapter 4). That is, while variation in user characteristics tends to mask the issue, there is an apparent trend for later studies evaluating the move to staffed housing (e.g. Bratt and Johnston, 1988; Mansell and Hughes, 1990) to fail to report the degree of benefit associated with initial or subsequent pilot or demonstration studies (e.g. Felce *et al.*, 1986; Mansell, 1994).

LONGER-TERM EFFECTS

Few studies have investigated the longer-term impact of deinstitutionalization. Those that have addressed this issue have tended to indicate a levelling off in the rate of improvement following the immediate move from institutional to community-based residential provision (e.g. Lowe and de Paiva, 1991; Cambridge *et al.*, 1994).

A number of factors may account for this phenomenon. Firstly, as noted above, evaluating change on the basis of informant reports may reflect changes in informant attitudes or expectations rather than changes in user behaviour. Thus, while changes in carer expectations may account for reported increases in challenging behaviour, they may also help explain, at least in part, some positive outcomes, for example, developments in adaptive behaviours. Secondly, the observed changes may simply reflect increased opportunities for participating in a range of activities in community-based settings. Thus, for example, increased proximity is likely to overcome some transportation barriers to participation in community-based activities. Similarly, devolved budgeting and the reduction in use of centralized purchasing and domestic services helps create readily accessible opportunities for participation in a wider range of domestic activities.

Whatever the reason for the plateau effect over time, it is readily apparent that there exists very little evidence that within community-based services users are developing new competencies, new relationships or extending the extent of their participation in their surrounding community over time.

COMPARATIVE AND NORMATIVE JUDGEMENTS

The majority of studies reviewed involved comparisons on a restricted range of outcome measures between two distinct models of service (Figure 11.2). While, at least more recently, it is apparent that this body of research has begun to incorporate some indicators of quality of life or lifestyle of service users (e.g. engagement, use of community-based facilities), some notable omissions continue to exist (cf. Emerson, 1985). In particular, little attention has been paid to the measurement of either broad social indicators of an individual's quality of life (e.g. wealth, disposable income, physical health, involvement in close and intimate personal relationships) or measurement of expressed life satisfaction. While the latter may, in part, reflect the severity of disability of some participants, such omissions are difficult to explain on the basis of technical difficulty or the resources required to collect such measures.

In addition, very few studies indeed involved normative judgements concerning the general adequacy, acceptability or decency of the quality of care provided or the quality of life experienced by people with learning disabilities in these settings (cf. Tøssebro, Chapter 5). Only one study in the current review incorporated comparisons between the lifestyle or quality of life of service users and non-disabled people (Stanley and Roy, 1988). This study reported similar levels of life satisfaction and overall quality of life but less use of community facilities reported by adults with learning disabilities compared to a group of non-disabled adults in the local community.

As a result, while the existing body of research may point to the overall superiority of new smaller community-based services over existing institutional provision, it offers little information which may help to form a broader judgement regarding the adequacy, acceptability or decency of the quality of life experienced by people with learning disabilities in these new settings. Answering this question must surely be reflected in any research agenda for the coming decade.

The transition to community services in Norway

12

Johans Sandvin

The social policy debate in Scandinavia is undergoing ideological changes. The traditionally strong support for the distinctive features of the Scandinavian welfare states, like equality, centralization, and universal social programmes, are gradually declining, and are being replaced by values that emphasize individual freedom and diversity, community and network, and decentralization of public services. There is growing political support for private and voluntary arrangements as alternatives to the public sector. These ideological changes are not merely Scandinavian phenomena. Decentralization and privatization have been general features in most western countries in the 1980s (Goldsmith and Newton, 1988; Kuhnle, 1990), and Communitarianism and the renaissance of the idea of Civil Society seem to be dominant ideologies in the 1990s (Bellah *et al.*, 1991; Seligman, 1992; Selznick, 1992; Coles, 1993; Etzioni, 1993).

Deinstitutionalization is another dominant feature in many western countries. Institution-based systems of care are being dismantled and replaced by ordinary housing or smaller residential homes in the community, following the guidelines of the principle of normalization and integration. Some of these changes are developing gradually, while others – requiring more structural change – are being channelled through public reforms.

In Norway one such reform concerns the care of people with developmental disabilities. From January 1991, the responsibility for providing services for people with developmental disabilities has been assigned to the local governmental authority (municipality or township), and the traditional institution-based system is rapidly being dismantled. This chapter gives a brief description of this reform and its implementation. Based on data from a recent survey of 72% of 440 Norwegian municipalities, a broad picture will be given of the service system that is about to be established locally. The reform will also be placed in a historical context, showing how the reform can throw light on some of the more general processes of the welfare state today.

THE CARE OF PEOPLE WITH DEVELOPMENTAL DISABILITIES IN NORWAY

In Norway, as in most western countries, the care of people with developmental disabilities has been dominated by institution-based care. In Norway, however, most of the institutions were established much later than in other western countries. In 1950 less than 1000 persons with developmental disabilities were receiving residential care in institutions. By 1970 this number had increased to more than 6000 (Chapter 5).

Already in the 1960s a rising tide of criticism of institutions in general made it difficult to continue institutional building, and in 1974 the government stated that care for people with developmental disabilities was the responsibility of local authorities. This ended any further expansion in institutional care, but did not enforce any activity from local authorities in establishing residential care for people in their home communities.

During the 1970s and 1980s the institutional care system was gradually restructured from large total institutions, to smaller institutions and residential homes. This change was, however, mainly carried out by the special health care service for people with developmental disabilities (called HVPU), at county level, which was responsible for the institutions, and not by local authorities.

Current estimates indicate that about 17 000 people with developmental disabilities need some form of public assistance in Norway. This represents slightly less than 0.4% of the population. Only about one-half receive any support from HVPU (one-third in institutional care). The other half have been the responsibility of local government, but very few services and supports have actually been provided locally.

THE REFORM

Today's reform includes not only a clear transfer of responsibility for service provision from county level to local authority level, but also a winding up of the HVPU and the institutions. Politically the reform is seen as one of the most important and far-reaching social reforms in Norway in the post-war period, the central goals of which are expressed by the concepts of normalization and integration. The quality of life for people with developmental disabilities should be brought to a level more equal to that of other citizens and should also include those people who did not receive any support from HVPU. To achieve these goals central government has issued rigid requirements for local preparation and planning prior to the transfer of responsibility, and the money which was previously spent by HVPU has been transferred to local authorities.

The significance of the Norwegian reform is, first of all, that it combines a total restructuring of the service system, with a decentralization of responsibility. Reform processes in other countries usually contain only one of these elements. Secondly, the Norwegian reform is total, in that it covers the whole country, while processes in many countries involves only counties, states or single institutions. The Norwegian reform is a demand made by central government which has put a lot of effort and prestige into it. Finally, the Norwegian reform is fast, with a reform period of five years. The final date for the closure of institutions was set for 1 January 1996, but of those 5000 people who were living in institutions when the reform came into force, more than 4000 had already moved out by the end of 1993.

The majority of people who have moved out of institutions have received services as stated in their individual plan. It also appears that the majority of the families are satisfied with the services offered, although there are still quite a number who feel disappointed. In a survey involving 241 families, 44% felt that the reform had led to a better supply of services; 38% felt that nothing had changed; while 8% felt that the provision of service had become poorer (Lund, 1992). The families of the previous HVPU users were the most satisfied which may imply that local authorities have, first of all, given priority to those who came from HVPU.

One significant reason for the positive follow-up local authorities have given the reform is the fact that they took over the financial responsibility for all developmentally disabled persons from 1 January 1991, including those who were still living in institutions. As people gradually moved out of institutions, the costs for those who still lived there constantly increased, thereby creating a financial incentive for local authorities to expedite the development of local services. In addition, the government, by exercising its right of appeal via the County Governor, has had the responsibility of postponing the transfer from institutions until adequate services were established in the municipalities. This has probably ensured a better provision of services than would have been the case had this right of appeal not existed. The standard of housing has also been influenced by the demands made by the Norwegian State Housing Bank.

The main problem for local authorities is that of the depressed state of the national economy and despite their own financial constraints are continuing to experience increased demand in commitment and expectations. Shortcomings in other areas of support is making it politically difficult for local authorities to give the reform the expected priority. There is also a big gap between the level of service required by law, and the ambitions and intentions in the reform which might affect the allocation of local resources when public attention around the reform reduces.

Nevertheless, even though there are obvious inadequacies in some places, and even though the future situation seems somewhat uncertain, it does look as though local authorities in general are capable of providing services which are at least as good as those provided by the institutional care system.

NORMALIZATION IMPLEMENTED?

The scope of service provision established by local authorities, however, tells us little about how the reform has contributed towards the realization of the more ideal intentions of the reform. We know that the majority of relatives of institution residents felt that the service provided by HVPU was satisfactory and did not need to be changed (Tøssebro, 1992b; Chapter 14). The fact that the majority of relatives of people who have moved from an HVPU institution are today satisfied, might in fact mean that, in reality, little has changed.

But the ambitions of the reform indicate something new: a realization of values that have developed over the past 20–25 years, based on a new perspective on people with developmental disabilities and a perspective that focuses more on common rights and needs of people in general, than on the special properties and limitations of people with developmental disabilities. To what extent, then, has the reform been able to realize its ideological agenda? To find the answer to such a question, we have to look not only at the scope of the services local authorities have established, but also at the form these services take. We shall point out some of the features we find to be fairly general.

More than half of those who previously lived in institutions are still living in the municipality where the institution is, or was situated, instead of moving back to the areas they originally came from. The care system in these municipalities is easily dominated by collective solutions which do not differ much from the care in institutions. There is a strong tendency towards standardized group housing which does not vary much from the houses built in connection with the restructuring of the institutional care system. Of the barely 6000 people who have been given new housing in the municipalities as a result of the reform, only 17% have been given individual, self-contained housing. In addition, 24% live in self-contained apartments, built together with other apartments for people with developmental disabilities. The remaining 60% have been given one form or another of collective housing. Of these, approximately one-half have a collective household. Of the municipalities where more than one collective housing scheme has been built, two-thirds have built terraced housing or detached housing on a site so that they form a natural unit. This can be advantageous with regard to resources such as staffing and surveillance, but features like the number of developmentally disabled residents, the shape and size of the houses and the number of employees, creates in many cases the distinctive impression of an institution.

This way of organizing housing easily leads to the need for rationalizing daily activities. Walks in the neighbourhood, barbecues on the lawn or organized transport to and from work or leisure activities easily become collective activities and create social distance from other neighbours and surroundings. There is also a greater temptation to build day-centres in connection with these houses, which increases the possibility for rational use of resources, but which also further emphasizes the impression of an institution.

During the planning stage, local authorities intended to integrate the provision of services for developmentally disabled people into the departments that provided equivalent services for other groups (Harsheim and Sandvin, 1991). However, it would appear that separate organizational units, especially for developmentally disabled people, have been established in the majority of municipalities (Sandvin, 1992). The Ministry of Social Welfare has warned against this in an official circular, but it seems that, among other reasons, the professions have a need to maintain the boundaries between the different service areas, in order to protect their technical domains.

At the same time, there are features which force a breaking down of these limits, and support the organizational coordination processes. The principles of both normalization and integration are used as arguments for removing the boundaries between service areas. Many local councils have recruitment difficulties and have to make use of the expertise available in the different areas of care provision. In addition, the ever more difficult economic situation in municipalities gives rise to the need for finding more rational forms of organization and operation and a more flexible use of personnel and skills.

This tendency is also apparent in the development of particular measures and services. Half of the municipalities have localized collective housing for people with developmental disabilities in connection with housing for the elderly or others in need of care, and approximately one-third have built collective housing in connection with health centres. All this can be advantageous with regard to personnel and supervision, but it can also lead to this form of housing being regarded more as a welfare measure than as private homes.

Although the reform is on schedule according to institutional closure and the establishment of local services, it has, to a lesser extent, been able to effect real changes in the content and profile of care. So far there is a general impression that the care system local authorities are in the process of establishing does not differ significantly from the care system that was to be replaced by the reform. Traditional institutions have been replaced by smaller houses of a higher material standard, situated closer to ordinary neighbourhoods, but still exhibiting clear features of being institutions. The institutional care system is disassembled, more than being dismantled. The most significant change in the municipal care system is that the differentiation between different groups and care measures is now less than was previously the case.

THE HISTORICAL AND POLITICAL CONTEXT

But the reform is not merely a question of restructuring a particular service system. The reform is a part of a much broader restructuring of the welfare state. Central values of the Scandinavian welfare state, such as public responsibility and standardized social programmes, are today being criticized for having created a colder society where people no longer feel responsible for each other; important social arenas like family, social networks and local communities are said to be 'crumbling' (Løchen, 1990). Decentralization and integration are seen as a means to reverse this process, and to restore 'gemeinschaft-relations' in society (Tönnies, 1912; Asplund, 1991). This vision is clearly expressed in the government White Paper:

> The reform is an important step towards a society for all, a society that does not push individuals or groups out of ordinary social life, but includes them in a fellowship of solidarity with mutual rights and duties.
>
> (St. meld. nr 67 1986–87. Author's translation).

The reform for people with developmental disabilities is but one of many reforms based on such values in Norway, and must be analysed in a broad social policy context.

DIFFERENTIATION

One way of gaining better understanding of the reform is to ask which values and concepts motivated the development of the care system that the reform is directed towards. What motivated the construction of the institution-based care system that the reform is about to dismantle?

The best place to search for the grounds and motivations behind the institutional system is probably in the National Plan for Care for the Mentally Retarded from 1952, and in the political debate that accompanied the plan. Here we can identify one concept that, more than any other, seems to characterize the ideas and assumptions in the social policy of that time. This concept was differentiation, formulated as a main principle for framing a new and comprehensive system of care. The plan talks about the need for: 'a comprehensive system of care for people with mental retardation [which] must first of all be based on special institutions, designed for people with mental retardation only ... consisting of several divided units or departments, designed for different purposes and categories of clients'.

During the latter part of the last century, developmentally disabled people were, to an increasing extent, separated from other institutional systems, such as special schools for the deaf and blind, asylums, and from ordinary schools. This differentiation formed the basis for special measures for developmentally disabled people, initially with schools and later nursing homes and residential training centres. At the beginning of this century, the developmentally disabled's movement was, to an increasing extent, dominated by medicine. The major idea behind the development of large regional institutions was the possibility of organizing differentiated medical and educational treatment, adjusted to the newer medical definition of developmental disability.

The development of the welfare state in general can also successfully be analysed in terms of differentiation. The post-war period was characterized by centralization, public expansion, and increased specialization, professionalization and sectorization. In all, the sector has more or less trebled its share of the gross national product from 1950 until the end of the 1970s. In 1980, 98 different occupational titles were registered within the health sector alone. Of these titles, 74 had arisen since the Second World War. The welfare state was a goal shared across political party lines, but the strong expansion in differentiation also developed its own motivating forces which were not always compatible with political aims – such as increased complexity, survey problems, problems connected with influence and availability – neither for those who were to use the welfare state nor for those who were to run it, and resulted in a sharp rise in costs.

But even before the financial problems became apparent, the welfare model demonstrated frictional problems. Criticism began to be directed towards the close concentration on economic growth and material prosperity which characterized welfare policy. Many people felt that the welfare state caused more problems than it solved. Terms like 'welfare problems' and 'welfare diseases' began to be used to describe families breaking up, juvenile crime, addiction and loneliness.

Furthermore, criticism was directed towards the ever increasing bureaucracy in the public sector which, it was claimed, was both inefficient and a threat to democracy. Concepts such as 'threshold', 'queue' and 'counter' were used to illustrate problems connected with accessibility, gaps between the services and the served, together with an unequal distribution of resources which characterized the welfare state's arrangements and reduced the accuracy of the social programmes. Bureaucratization was also criticized for reducing the effect of increased access to resources. The growth led to more jobs in the welfare sectors rather than increasing the welfare of the users.

The third and ultimately the most important criticism was directed towards the heavy pressure on costs, caused by the developments in welfare. The stable economic growth throughout the 1950s and 1960s was replaced, in the 1970s, by the poor trade outlook in Europe – conditions which eventually also reached Norway. This led to greater attention being paid to the increasing growth in the public sector and brought about strong demands for a more efficient organization of the welfare state and a reduction in public spending.

Steering an ever more specialized and differentiated society also led to the need for specialized and differentiated expertise in public administration, and the transfer of significant power and autonomy to the bureaucracy. This development was characterized in Norway by differentiation and greater autonomy in administrative units, both in internal public administration and through the establishing of free-standing directorates. The planning and initiating of public policy presupposed an ever closer cooperation with organized social interests, and changed the traditional patterns of interaction and conflict within society; the 'negotiating state' is a concept which illustrates this development (Olsen, 1988).

But the close integration in the governing system, both between levels in the public sector and between the public sector and organized interests, created problems. The increasing sectorization led to problems with coordination and democracy; differences in organizational resources between different social groups and interests maintained or increased social inequality. Integration also created an organizational rigidity which turned processes of restructuring and change into heavy negotiation processes, with a lot of conflict. In addition, the integration model caused a sharp rise in costs because its legitimacy was based on the concept that everyone realized their own interests. The government's ability to govern according to overall national interests gradually decreased and became dependent on continuing economic growth. Tighter economic conditions since the end of the 1970s, and an increasing political demand for efficiency, created the need for an extensive reorganization of public administration to ensure a stricter general financial steering.

TOWARDS DEDIFFERENTIATION

A major reform programme for the 'modernization' of the public sector was started at the beginning of the 1980s. The market was to become less regulated; laws were to be simplified; special laws were to be replaced by a more open framework of law, and all were to be given greater freedom.

Among the most important measures is decentralization of responsibility to a lower level of decision-making and a number of such reforms have already seen the light of day. In many ways, the decentralization policy of the 1980s can be regarded as a return of tasks and responsibility to local authority level. Symbols like nearness, network, community and informal care indicate that there is a desire to recreate some of the local social qualities that disappeared as a result of the expansion of the welfare state. Decentralization of tasks and responsibility to local authority level emerge as an important strategy for realizing such a policy.

The processes of change in social policy during the 1980s, such as decentralization, debureaucratization, deregulation and deprofessionalization, must be interpreted as anti-processes to the differentiation and complexity which characterize the modern treatment society.

The major features of the criticism of institutions and in the development of the normalization ideology, is the reversal of the differentiation which characterized the start of care for developmentally disabled people. The development follows the same course as the differentiation, only in reversed order. The differentiation started with the definition of developmentally disabled people as a group, independent of other groups. This formed the basis for the establishment of new offers of care specially directed towards people with developmental disabilities – first schools and then nursing homes. After medicine began to dominate the care system, we experienced an increasing differentiation within the care system, and the establishment of the large institutions, where differentiation was an explicit principle of organization.

While this differentiation was based on the distinctive characteristics of developmentally disabled people, and on the differences within the category with regard to intelligence, level of functioning and diagnosis, normalization ideology focused on handicapped people as human beings in general, and on the similarities between people with and without handi-

caps. The claim was first that life within the institution had to be organized in a way as similar as possible to life in the outside world. Criticism
was later directed more towards the physical differentiation that the institutions represented. The institutions themselves were defined as the
major problem. Today, the ideology of normalization is more and more
often directed towards the very definition of developmentally disabled
people as a distinctive group or category, in other words, towards the
very foundation for the establishment of a special care system.

The ideology of normalization is – as the concept itself indicates – an
ideology of dedifferentiation. The major elements of the concept are
equality and integration, while the main elements of differentiation are
inequality and separation. The policy of normalization and integration
are closely connected to the general criticism of the welfare state. The
political and ideological processes that have taken place in the rest of
social policy and in politics in general, such as deregulation, decentralization and deinstitutionalization in favour of a stronger belief in family, network and community, created quite another political climate for a care
system reform.

Thus, the Norwegian reform does not emerge as an isolated phenomenon created by consumer organizations and ideologists, but as part of a
far more general reform programme. And the ideology of normalization
and integration represents a definite ideological expression of values
which had far more general roots. It expressed growing scepticism
towards the traditional welfare state's formal, specialized solutions,
towards the planned economy and large-scale arrangements, and
towards social engineering's organizational building and breaking up of
the close relationships we associate with the old rural society.
Normalization, and integration, were ideological expressions of a general
dedifferentiation ideology.

Taking another look at some of the features of the care system that
local authorities have so far established for people with developmental
disabilities to replace the institutional care, we feel that much of what
local authorities today call integration is more in accordance with what
we have called dedifferentiation. People who had previously received
care within the special health service for developmentally disabled people
(HVPU), today receive services from a care system which also provides
services for other groups of handicapped people. Houses for people with
developmental disabilities are built in a number of municipalities in connection to houses for other people requiring assistance or in connection to
service centres with an extended system of help. Almost one-third of the
municipal day-centres that have been established in connection with the
reform are also used by people who are not developmentally disabled –

very often people with psychiatric problems, and a number of older people with developmental disabilities (who aren't always so old) are placed in ordinary old people's homes. The intention is that people with developmental disabilities are to be treated in the same way as all others who are in need of assistance, not as a special group. This represents a clear dedifferentiation, a reversal of the differentiation process which began by defining the developmentally disabled as a target group – and ended up establishing large special institutions. At the same time an important motivating force for this differentiation was to separate people with developmental disabilities from other assistance arrangements. The policy today is to make arrangements for public assistance as general as possible.

CONCLUSION

Summing up the discussion we can conclude that the Norwegian reform for people with developmental disabilities is not the pitfall that the defenders of the old system claimed it would be. Norwegian municipalities have shown that they are capable of providing services for people with developmental disabilities that are at least as good as the service provided by the county council, and most of the criticism has disappeared. But the lack of criticism also conceals that little has in fact changed. The structure of the service system has changed, but the content of the care remains more or less the same – it is only provided on a smaller scale. The history of the Norwegian reform so far – being a success in many ways – is a history not of dissolution of institutions, but more of disassembling of institutional care – and of reintegration on a lower level of differentiation.

To what extent the ideals and intentions of the reform – in particular the ideals of social integration – are possible to achieve is difficult to say. One of the problems with the Norwegian reform is that it seems more reactive than proactive; instead of actively seeking new solutions, the old ones seem to be reversed. Instead of establishing comprehensive support for living in a modern differentiated society, the government hopes for a recreation of a society of the past, with homogeneous and socially integrated local communities.

But this hope rests upon a rather unrealistic picture of local communities. The ideal type of local community has probably never existed in its pure form, and today it has even lost most of its previous characteristics. Most people live in cities or urban areas. Modern life, with all that it consists of, has reached even the smallest and most remote communities. The places where people used to meet, like the local post office, the local general store, the quay, or the church or prayer house have either disappeared or lost their previous functions. Social patterns do not follow geographical or residential patterns, and social networks are based more on work, education, lifestyle and personal choice, than on neighbourhood or kinship. The Norwegian reform, which reflects the criticism of institutions and segregation, seems to imply the belief that when the impersonal and controlling institutional structures are removed, a natural, informal and caring community is automatically regained.

These processes also correspond with more general processes in the welfare state. In fact the reform illustrates very well the features of change that characterize the present social policy in general, ideologically as well as organizationally. Organizationally the social policy can be described as a process of dedifferentiation; a reactive response to the problems of differentiation, guided by goals and ambitions that go far beyond the limits of politics.

PART FOUR:
The Impact on Families of Service Users

Relatives' opinions on institutional closure 13

Barbro Tuvesson and Kent Ericsson

In this chapter, the process of moving away from the institutional tradition in the provision of support to people with intellectual handicaps is illustrated by a project carried out in the County of Skaraborg. In this county institutional care had been established very early. Emanuella Carlbeck, the woman who established the first institution for people with handicaps lived in this county, and the residential institution which she founded was regarded as a model institution for a long period, not just in this county but throughout the country.

The shift away from institutional care started in the first half of the 1970s when the early community services began to develop, a process which continued throughout the 1970s and 1980s. When the 1985 Act came into force, stipulating that institutions were no longer an acceptable way of providing support and service, a decision was taken to close down the three residential homes in the county. Three hundred people were affected by this decision and by the ensuing process of change, which took place during the second half of the 1980s.

As explained in Chapter 6, when state support for people with intellectual handicaps was endorsed in 1954, a centralized organization for special services was established. This was run by the county administration, which was given the task of providing special support through services for which they were directly responsible. This relieved all other authorities in society from any responsibility for this group. In addition to the closure of institutions, the powers and responsibilities of this centralized special organization are being devolved to municipal authorities. People with intellectual handicaps are instead being given access to the support which is provided by organizations responsible for providing service to the general public. For example, in relation to housing, the municipal authority responsible for public housing for others is now also responsible for housing for this group. As a consequence the county authority is being dissolved in accordance with the development of the capacity and competence of the municipalities to meet the needs of people with intellectual disabilities.

In the County of Skaraborg, with 17 local municipal authorities, the change from a centralized special service organization had already begun when work started on the replacement of institutional care with community services. This meant that 17 persons, one in each of the municipalities, were given the key role in this process of change, their task being to create alternative services to which residents were to move (Ericsson, 1994).

A CHANGE IN THE ROLE OF THE FAMILY

In the miniature society created within the institution the objective was to take complete care of the people with intellectual handicaps who lived there. Everything that they needed should be available there. Other organizations were not expected to take responsibility, this being a stipulated duty for the county authority (Ericsson, 1993). This view of responsibility and resources for people with intellectual handicaps was reflected also in relations with their families. When the person was admitted to the institution his family, parents, siblings and others, were not expected to assume any responsibility for their care or welfare. The location of these (often regionally sited) institutions also contributed to making contact more difficult. Initially visiting hours and times were also closely regulated, only being allowed at certain times. Such limitations contributed to difficulties in maintaining normal relationships between families and relatives at the institution.

This tradition has been established for a long time and has therefore had a strong impact on this field of care. New ideas concerning a more normal life, and an integration of the support provided, have gradually evolved in Sweden and have now developed so far that community services are those now considered most desirable.

Relatives, on the contrary, are not responsible for the services provided by society. For them it is contact with their son or daughter at the institution which is the pertinent issue. When, therefore, notification came saying that the institution was to be closed down, they were faced with an entirely new situation. Within a short period they were confronted with a new ideology, and newly-developed services. They were also faced with an entirely new future for their son or daughter and thereby for the entire family. Where information is lacking as to the nature of the alternative service which is to replace the institution, a decision to close down the institution will appear as illogical. The family is well aware that their relative is in need of support and service. It is therefore easy to fear that they will no longer receive support of any kind if the institution is closed down. When the relatives are informed that the institution will be closed it is not uncommon that the reaction is one of anxiety, even anger and aggression. Families are suddenly faced with new circumstances which can totally change their life – that of the person being cared for at the institution and that of the family themselves. Nor need it be the case in this situation that, as a relative, one believes all one is told. Instead the family may have their own experience to draw on. At the time when their child was originally placed at the institution, the decision often led to a life of very simple, meagre and, at times, even destructive conditions, regardless of what had been promised.

These views can change during the process which takes place while the institution is undergoing closure. People move to new and more modern services. If these are found to be better for the person, then it is probable that they will also be contented with the new life. For relatives closure will be a question of what consequences will be incurred, and the nature of these changes will be reflected in the views and experiences of the relatives (Ericsson, 1987b). An overall interest in how relatives perceive the change from institutional to community services therefore lies behind this study. It is concerned with the issue of how relatives understand and react to the process of deinstitutionalization which their family members have experienced (Ericsson, 1994; Tuvesson, 1994).

INTERVIEWS WITH RELATIVES

Relatives of those who had left a large residential institution were asked about their attitude towards the closure of the institution. In all, interviews were carried out with 53 relatives, representing 36 people who had moved. Of these relatives 28 were parents, 14 sisters and brothers and 11 were related in other ways. In 18 interviews one relative was met, while in the rest two or three people participated. Most often they were husbands and wives, but there were also sisters and brothers together with other relatives. At the time of the interview, the intellectually disabled relative had been out of the institution for a period of one to four years.

The aim of the interview was to learn what relatives thought of the information they had received about the closure of the institution and to ask them to assess the new conditions, in order to evaluate whether they had kept or changed their early views. The first subject was relatives' reactions to the early information they received about the closure. The question to these relatives was: 'When you were informed about the closure of the institution, what did you think?' Secondly, relatives were asked about the new conditions offered through the community services to which they had moved. They were asked to describe and comment on the new conditions, based upon their views of the home of their disabled relative. The interviews were semi-structured: relatives talked freely while answering the questions during the interview. With the help of notes and tape recordings, an opinion was formed using the comments of the relatives; these were then grouped into three broad categories – positive, negative and neutral.

Table 13.1 The opinion of relatives before and after the move from the institution

Before	After			Sum
	negative	neutral	positive	
Negative	2	4	9	15
Neutral	1	1	9	11
Positive	–	–	10	10
Sum	3	5	28	36

Table 13.1 summarizes the views of relatives before and after the move from the institution. The relatives of ten persons were positive about institutional closure before it happened and those ten are still positive after the move has taken place. Of the 15 interviews where the relatives were initially negative, two are still negative after the move, four have become neutral and nine now have a positive attitude. Among the 11 with neutral views before, nine have become positive. One person is still neutral and one has changed from a neutral to a negative opinion – the only one among the 36 interviews where there was a change in a negative direction.

RELATIVES' VIEWS ABOUT INSTITUTIONAL CLOSURE

POSITIVE REACTIONS TO THE INITIAL INFORMATION

'I was the first to telephone and apply for him', an elderly mother said. When she got the information that the institution was to close, she telephoned and applied for a group home in her community for her son. He usually stayed with her every weekend, was always upset on Sunday nights when he was due to go back to the institution his mother saw the opportunity to change this. There were other parents in a similar situation. There had been upsetting farewells, and because of that parents had not seen their children as often as they had wanted to. To these parents the closure of the institution was a welcomed change. They had nothing to lose.

'I thought it would be better for him. Freer. I was never an opponent', said one brother. One sister said she had a bad conscience during all the years her brother spent at the institution. When she was in her twenties and he was ten years old, her parents were given the ultimatum of either employing a tutor for their son or sending him to a residential school. Even today his sister is in tears when she talks about that situation. Her parents were working-class people and could not possibly employ a teacher so her brother was sent to the institution and has been there ever since. Through this institutional closure the sister saw the opportunity for rehabilitation. Other relatives, also positive about the change, thought that a new way of living could have far-reaching consequences. Their disabled relatives would get their freedom and would be spared isolation.

'I will never forget', one mother said, 'the headmaster who said that my son had to go to the residential school in order to learn something. That was plain speaking. It was horrible. He was only ten years old'. She had had trouble throughout the years because her son would often lay down in the hall and scream when he didn't want to return to the institution. When she received the information that the institution was to be closed, she thought things would improve.

Although we did not specifically ask relatives about their experiences when leaving their son or daughter at the institution for the first time, seven of the 36 talked about it anyway. They remembered receiving a letter, or information from a doctor or a headmaster, and they could still present the information literally. Of the seven who talked about this, five were positive when they got the information about the closure of the institution.

NEGATIVE REACTIONS TO THE INITIAL INFORMATION

To some people the information came as a shock as they thought they had their relatives safely placed at a residential institution with competent staff 24 hours a day and counted on them staying there indefinitely. 'It was horrible', two elderly parents said. 'We were totally taken by surprise, and so were the rest of the parents, at least those who said something'. 'The information came as if someone poured cold water over me'. 'How will it be?' 'Will it work?' 'It will never work for him to move back home again.'

Many people feared their relatives would get less help in the future. 'It won't work', two parents said, 'he cannot cook for himself'. Representatives for the county authorities talked about people having 'their own apartments in the home community'. The families thought that their relatives would be sitting alone in apartments, with little or no support from staff.

These apartments would be in the home community of the families and their conclusion was that they would be expected to resume full responsibility. One brother, in fear of this, said afterwards, 'I never thought they would spend so much money on the intellectually handicapped'. He was opposed to the closure but he had also been negative to the institution. 'If one is healthy moving into such a corridor, then one isn't well moving out'.

Other relatives who were negative about the move said it was foolish to move a person who was rooted in an environment where they seemed to be happy. 'They were so settled there. They had a church and everything, and then they would have to adjust to something new'.

Thus the relatives who were negative about the institutional closure had different reasons; some wanted things to stay the same and others felt worried about the impending changes.

NEUTRAL REACTIONS TO THE INITIAL INFORMATION

Other relatives reacted neither positively nor negatively as they could see both the advantages and disadvantages for the move and despite reservations about the quality of support that would be available, they didn't want to stop the development. 'If it influences them in the right direction, then it is right', one mother said. 'Perhaps I heaved a sigh of relief that he was going to be his own master', one sister said. 'We were worried, but wanted to wait and see; we wouldn't stop it', two parents said. 'We didn't think so much about it as it wouldn't happen all at the same time', one sister told me. She had seen her brother being mistreated when, early in his life, he had stayed with different farmers. When he at last came to the institution that difficult period was over. The move from the institution to a supported apartment was not that dramatic. Two parents said: 'It is hard to compare an apartment with the residential institution. There is a bigger difference between being home and being at an institution'.

A CHANGE FROM A NEGATIVE OR NEUTRAL TO A POSITIVE OPINION

Many of those, who changed to a more positive view, said they did this shortly after the move. When they could actually see that their disabled relatives had adjusted to the new life and seemed to be happy, they changed their minds and considered the new service as something positive. 'We changed opinions almost at once. It was easy to see the quality in the apartments', said two parents.

Some relatives said they changed their opinion before the move, in response to the information given, for example, when shown the place where staff were to be based, or in response to promises made about the improved standard of care for the disabled relatives. 'At first I was hesitant and thought that she would end up in the middle of town, not being able to move about. Then I got to see the grounds and the drawings of the new house, and I was delighted and understood this was really something extra', one mother siad. 'When there was a decision made that she was to eat in the dining-room and be helped every day, then I thought that this would work out well', said a relative of a woman who moved into a supported apartment.

A CHANGE FROM A NEGATIVE TO A NEUTRAL OPINION

The relatives who were negative before the move, and neutral afterwards, could see that the new life provided advantages which they hadn't expected. But they also thought there were some things missing. An elderly mother, living in a small place, thinks it is great to have her son back home. He lives in a group home within ten minutes walking distance from her. They meet several days a week, which she appreciates. However, she is disappointed that he is not getting the same quality of care he received at the institution. There are enough staff, but she is dissatisfied with their achievements. 'Nobody takes responsibility', she says. Some parents are worried about the staff's medical competence, for example, in dealing with epilepsy. 'To the staff it is safe that we live nearby. We are more acquainted with the boy than a doctor is. It is hard for the staff to know when to call for a doctor', two parents said.

One mother who was negative before and is now neutral, described her experiences like this: 'At the institution they took care of my worries. These worries have come closer now, and that is both positive and negative'.

A CHANGE FROM A NEUTRAL TO A NEGATIVE OPINION

At one interview we met relatives who saw the move as a deterioration. They were two sisters who were neutral to the move, but afterwards viewed it as negative. They described their brother as having a 'diminished world' as he now had fewer friends with no real relationships and his constant state of agitation and restlessness had become a major concern.

CONFIRMING A POSITIVE OPINION

For the ten individual people who were positive before the move, and continued to be positive afterwards, the measures taken had, as expected, resulted in improved conditions. Those people visiting their relatives no longer needed to undertake long, arduous journeys; parents were able to re-establish regular fortnightly problem-free visits with their relatives and relatives now quite readily returned to their own community-based housing. As a result of this increased freedom parents were able to experience their son or daughter developing as a person. 'We are most happy for his sake,' one father said. 'They were so isolated at the institution.'

CONFIRMING A NEGATIVE OPINION

Among the 15 negative interviews at the early stage, two were still negative after the move. One interview was about a woman in her seventies who moved to a home for the elderly. Her relatives felt that she had been sent to the wrong place. 'There are too few staff. She is just sitting there, and does not get activated. The staff think we should take part and we don't have the time'. The woman had become unruly, and the staff could not always handle her, they would telephone the relatives and ask them to come and help.

In the other instance parents spoke of their son who lives in his own apartment, and is cared for and nursed by staff at home. The son receives visiting support five times a day, and in spite of this they felt that he was undernourished, unkempt and his place was in a mess. He has epilepsy, and on one occasion the hospital telephoned them to say that he had been admitted a few days ago and that as parents they had to answer for his poor hygiene. 'There were stockings "standing for themselves" and long-johns that stank. Do you understand how it feels being a mother and having to stand this when he has so many staff around him?'

The parents obviously felt that the support he was receiving was inadequate and despite the availability of staff his needs were not met. This couple had been most worried about the move. They felt that the root of the problem lay in raising his expectations, with regard to the extent of his personal freedom, prior to the move, without introducing the opportunity to undertake effective whole-environment post-transfer training.

CONFIRMING A NEUTRAL OPINION

One interview involved relatives who were neutral after as well as before the move. They couldn't remember their initial reaction to the information, however, they do remember it was their sister herself telling them that she was going to move. They think it is good for her to have an apartment of her own where she can be her own mistress. However, they don't like the fact that the apartment is situated in a noisy area and are worried that she will get into bad company. They also think that she feels lonely sometimes, which she denies.

DISCUSSION

There is one question to which an immediate answer has been provided by this study. This is the question of whether the families who to begin with had negative expectations regarding the changes taking place, were still negative in their views after the person had moved. The answer was that the majority of this group had changed their opinions so that now most were positive about what had taken place. Whereas 28% had been positive before the outset of the move, 78% were positive afterwards. There is, therefore, a group who have changed their point of view after being able to see the alternatives being offered and experience the new life which has been made available to their relative.

But there is also a group who, in spite of the new services which have been developed, are not entirely satisfied with what is being provided. They are, admittedly, a small group but they are not content even if the material and formal conditions are of a high standard. When they view the alternatives they see other qualities as important in order to regard the service as suitable for their relative. One conclusion to be drawn from this is that it is not always enough that the new forms of service created meet the formal and material demands and requirements, it is also important to have the assurance that these criteria are also considered important by others, in particular by the family. If one is interested in understanding their point of view it is necessary that they be involved and participate in the process of change, and be given an opportunity to influence the type of life their sons or daughters are going to live.

The closer proximity between the person and his family, brought about by the process of change, has been important. Although not everyone lives nearer their family, many live much closer to each other than previously. This has created the opportunity for the development of a completely new type of relationship between the person and his family. Prior to this, formal contact could be maintained but was often associated with long journeys and visits to an unfamiliar environment at the institution. This has been replaced by the possibility of meeting each under more informal and spontaneous circumstances and in familiar everyday situations. There are, admittedly, families who expressed a wish not to have their relative living in the same municipality as themselves. And there are still people who do not live near their families. Considering these results one can ask why they have not been given this opportunity.

A significant impression from this study is the very strong bond between the family and their relative. They are seen as an integral part of the family, and these families live with the intellectually disabled relative even if he or she is not always physically present. Families view the change which has taken place from a life-long perspective and the person is clearly in their thoughts even if they have been away and it has not been possible to share or influence their lives for many decades. Decisions about institutional placement which took place long ago are still well remembered.

The commitment shown here indicates the role of the family and the responsibility family members feel for their handicapped relative, even if that person has not always been part of their everyday life. This is an expression of the person belonging to a family. For the organization responsible for providing support and services this is an important assertion. The person who is intellectually handicapped does not 'belong' to the organization and need not be subjected to the measures which they consider should be taken. Of course, as a provider of the services offered by society, it has an important role to play in relation to people with intellectual handicaps. But whilst making decisions on proposals and measures to be taken, it also infringes on the lives of families in ways which can influence them dramatically. The closure of the institution and the residents' move to new forms of support and service is an example of such a measure.

Family attitudes to deinstitutionalization in Norway

14

Jan Tøssebro

My point of departure is a puzzle. On the one hand, institutions for people with mental retardation have been criticized for years, and principles like 'integration' and 'normalization' are approved by politicians, professionals and parents' societies. When the Norwegian parliament decided to dismantle residential institutions for people with mental retardation, it actually enshrined in law support for the view that institutions are not fit places in which to live. The parents' society had strongly advocated this reform.

On the other hand, reports of opposing or anxious parents are a frequent occurrence in the newspapers. They tell a story of coercive relocation; of parents' wishes being overridden by the authorities. As I will show, there is no reason to doubt that the image created by the media is accurate, and neither is this parental opposition a phenomenon special to Norway. North American findings indicate that a large majority of parents are opposing deinstitutionalization (66%–83%, Meyer, 1980; Landesman-Dwyer, 1981; Heller *et al.*, 1988; Latib *et al.*, 1984; Larson and Lakin, 1991) and there is a strong British lobby opposing closure (Chapter 15).

Hence the puzzle: a social reform, which is supported as progressive and enlightened by the parental society and the policy community, is regarded as a threat by ordinary parents. This paper will present some details on family opposition in Norway, but attention will primarily be paid to the explanation of why ordinary parents oppose deinstitutionalization.

DATA

The data presented in this chapter was provided by postal questionnaires obtained from 484 relatives, most of them parents (65% of respondents were parents, 28% siblings and 7% other relatives; for simplicity, I will call them parents), and telephone calls to about 40 people. The data were gathered as a supplement to the survey on living conditions in mental retardation institutions referred to in Chapter 5. The questionnaire was mailed to 571 persons who had accepted participation in the living conditions survey (where staff were interviewed). The response rate was 84.8% (64.2% of those not accepting participation in the living condition survey are included). Non-respondents do not seem to differ much from respondents, though there is a slight under-representation of parents of residents over 50 in one of the counties. The data are probably fairly representative nationally. One problem with the data is, however, worth mentioning: the number of unanswered questions is rather high on questions where knowledge on life in the institution was required (details in Tøssebro, 1990b). It is also important to note that the respondents are not representing parents of all Norwegians with mental retardation, only the one-third living in institutions. Parents of those living at home express views moderately favourable to the deinstitutionalization programme.

The people spoken to by telephone were by no means randomly selected. They selected themselves. When we wrote to parents to get permission for interviews in the institution, some ticked the option for more information. I telephoned these individuals, and the conversation quickly switched from our study to their opinion, experience and uneasiness. They were far from representative, but conversations with them turned out to be important to the interpretation of survey data.

The telephone calls and gathering of survey data took place at a time when uneasiness concerning the implementation of deinstitutionalization reached a peak (Autumn 1989–Spring 1990). The findings are to be interpreted in such a context, and generalizations to other contexts should be cautious.

ATTITUDES OF NORWEGIAN PARENTS TO DEINSTITUTIONALIZATION

Table 14.1 shows extensive scepticism about the proposed closure. No more than 15% believed the Ministry's promise of improvement. Nearly two-thirds expected worsening conditions. These figures are in keeping with the proportion opposing deinstitutionalization in North America (Meyer, 1980; Landesman-Dwyer, 1981; Heller et al., 1988; Larson and Lakin, 1991; Latib et al., 1984).

Two comments made by parents who telephoned illustrate the degree of concern:

Table 14.1 Do you think the person you are related to will be offered improved conditions when the local authorities take over?

	%
Yes, sure	4
Yes, probably	11
Makes no difference	23
No, the institutions were better	44
No, this will all go wrong	18
Total	100
N	391

Missing cases/do not know: 18% of 484.

> 'You cannot relocate him. You are turning me into a nervous wreck. You know he will be troublesome if relocated. Why are you doing this?'; and 'This is horrible – sending letters about relocation of the children. Parents are supposed to decide for their children. Such letters open old wounds; the retarded will never be normal. This has gone much too far. Stop it instead of sending such letters'.

A range of other questions confirms the distribution shown in Table 14.1: 44% disagree with the statement 'I feel secure and informed about what is happening', 59% agree that 'parents will now have to take too large a part in the care', and 72% agree that 'local authorities are too ignorant on mental retardation to do the job properly'. Answers to these kind of questions are strongly correlated ($r=0.36$ to 0.48, factor loadings 0.72 to 0.73 on the same factor after principal component analysis and varimax rotation), probably reflecting an underlying attitude: extent of uneasiness and opposition.

Only a small minority welcomed the reform, but the extensive opposition does not necessarily mean a hostile attitude to principles like normalization. Worries about current changes do not imply support for past ideology: that people with mental retardation are best off if protected in residential institutions. To obtain a more subtle picture of their attitudes, respondents were presented with a series of statements, among which they were asked to pick the two best expressing their own opinion.

Table 14.2 also shows only minor support for the reform. Only 10% ticked the statement expressing unambiguous support (this compares

Table 14.2 Family attitudes to deinstitutionalization

	First reply (%)	Second reply (%)	Total (%)
It is positive, and time the institutions were dismantled and the generic service system takes responsibility	9	1	10
It is a good idea, but I am afraid the implementation will be poor	27	11	38
It is a good idea, but it should not include all. Some need the institutions	31	18	49
It is a good idea, but residents who have been living there for a long time should be allowed to stay. New entrants should, however, be prohibited	10	14	24
Improvement of institutions would have been a better option	9	13	22
The institutions provide quality care, and this reform ought to be stopped before it is too late	3	6	9
No response	11	37	–
Total	100	100	–
N	484	484	–

Each respondent could tick two statements. First reply is not assumed to be more important than the second.

with 21% of parents of people living in the family home). Neither was support for the institutions very frequent as 9% wanted to stop the dismantling, and 22% preferred continuation of the improvement of institutions. Most of the respondents preferred the ambiguous statements – expressing support for the principle of normalization, but opposition to total dismantling and doubts with respect to the ongoing implementation.

It seems reasonable to interpret these data like this: a group of people, deeply concerned about the well-being of people with mental retardation, regarded the reform as wishful thinking that could turn into a threat: 'The best is the enemy of the good'. Or, as one father expressed it: 'This ship of ideology is about to crush the one haven we have got'.

Why should there be this negative attitude to a social reform advocated by the parental society as the one route to progress? I will pay atten-tion to two broad issues. Firstly, it seems that one important problem is anxiety about what is to happen. Research has shown that in general atti-tudes become more positive after the relocation has taken place (Larson and Lakin, 1991; Landesman-Dwyer, 1981; Heller *et al.*, 1988; Chapter 13), and it is quite possible that involvement in planning of the new services and housing would affect attitudes in about the same way. Part of the problem could be that alternatives to institutions are rather vague before people have experience of them.

Secondly, it seems that ordinary parents find the contemporary institu-tions satisfactory, and consequently, deinstitutionalization appears as an unnecessary and risky venture. Before going on, however, it is important to refute a hypothesis about parental opposition that is frequently heard among Norwegian professionals. It is often suggested that the primary concern of the parents' society is people with a milder mental retardation, while opposition to deinstitutionalization is more frequent among par-ents of severely retarded persons. This is out of keeping with the data. No correlation exists between parents' attitudes and severity of handicap.

THE UNCLEAR ALTERNATIVE

I was rather surprised when I asked parents' permission to interview staff on living conditions in the institutions, and about 20% ticked the option for 'more information wanted'. The surprise did not diminish after the first telephone calls: the parents did not want information on the research at all, but were confused that someone bothered to ask their permission. The information they wanted was personal: 'Do you know what is going to happen to my son/daughter?' They knew about the reform, but next to nothing about the practical implications for the one they cared for: 'Is she going to be relocated?' 'Where is she going to live?'

This uneasiness was not without foundation. The organization respon-sible for residential services was going to disappear. Other organizations, i.e. the local authorities, who had never done much for people with men-tal retardation (less than their legal obligations), were to be solely respon-sible. Furthermore, the media image of the local authorities is of continuous fiscal crisis, and poor services for people needing public care, i.e. the elderly. Fiscal problems were also the focus of attention in the public debate on deinstitutionalization. Late clarification concerning the economic transfers from central to local government produced uncer-tainty, and this was passed on to parents, partly through a media game where local authorities insisted that the reform was going to be a disaster unless more money were transferred, and partly because local authorities hesitated to inform people about the ongoing planning: 'First things first – we need economic clarification before we can say anything definite'.

It could be argued that county authorities, formerly responsible for residential services for people with mental retardation, have a fiscal crisis of their own, and the mass media have not been silent about this. Such an objection, however, misses the important point. Parents have real experiences with the institutional system – they know what they have got. The question is whether they know what they will get. Principles like 'normalization' and 'integration' may sound right, but the parents' concern is: 'about the consequences for their children'. Reference to principles is not a satisfactory reply as principles sound more like wishful thinking. Realistic, materialized visions are wanted, but good examples from elsewhere are not particularly reassuring when your own community has done next to nothing.

In order to make the alternative look more realistic, one option is to involve parents in planning. This could be done by participation, or by providing sufficient information to permit parents to place their trust in public services. The ministry presupposed such participation, at least with respect to the individual need assessment plans (which were a mandatory part of the deinstitutionalization process) (Ot. prp. (Parliamentary Bill) 49, 1987–88, for example p.16).

The data show that for most parents, involvement in planning could not possibly have made the alternatives to the institutional care less vague. Table 14.3 shows low perceived levels of influence, and Table 14.4 that the plans are still unclear – about eight months prior to the start of implementation. The lack of clarity may reflect poor information or that plans were still vague; most likely both. Whatever the reasons, only a minority of parents were presented a satisfactory basis for trust. Tables 14.3 and 14.4 are examples from a wider range of questions, all correlated (correlations 0.29–0.46, loading 0.65–0.74 on the same factor in factor analysis after principal component analysis and varimax rotation) and pointing in the same direction. Most parents were distant from the planning, though exceptions obviously occurred.

Taken together, the questions on information and participation indicate that parents can be classified in three groups of about equal size. First, some parents regard themselves as having next to no influence and they have not been presented with anything down to earth on the alternative to the institution. The next third consists of those who have been asked their opinion as a part of the planning process, or have been to information meetings. The last group includes those who can see the outline of the new services. In the tables to come, these three groups are

Table 14.3 In your opinion, did you have any say in the planning of new services to the person you are related to?

	%
No, not at all	45
No, and we did not want to get involved	6
Yes, some influence	32
Yes, the authorities have largely taken our opinion into account	17
Total	100
N	477

Table 14.4 Do you know how the plans concerning the person you are related to are progressing?

	%
Do not know	24
Plans are still vague	31
Plans are beginning to take shape	20
Planning has come far	20
It is ready for relocation	5
Total	100
N	479

called spectators, by-standers and participants on a composite measure of unclearness.

The parents have characteristics which frequently go with shortage of political and administrative resources. Most of the parents were elderly, and usually deceased when siblings or other relatives answered the questionnaire. In the group of respondents (parents, siblings and other family) 52% were over 60 years old, 44% were retired and 71% did not have secondary education. This, however, does not seem to have affected participation in the planning process. The parents' social and economic situation does not explain the variance. The number of residents in the institution, however, has a certain impact. About 50% of the parents of residents in small institutions (less than 25 residents), can be classified as participants. The corresponding figure on large institutions is 25%. This is probably straightforward to explain: in small institutions, parents are likely to be in touch with management, who presumably are well-informed. In large institutions, contacts are likely to be with nursing staff or the ward supervisor at best. The correlation between size and unclearness cannot be explained by the small institutions being converted into new permanent housing since this also occurred with some large institutions.

The assumption of this section has been that the unclearness of the alternative affects attitudes to deinstitutionalization. Table 14.5 shows that such is the case. The correlation between the two variables is 0.34. It is worth noting that in the two non-participating groups, about two-thirds are negative or hostile to deinstitutionalization. The corresponding figure among the participants is one-third. Consequently, there is reason to believe that opposition and hostility could be substantially reduced by involving parents.

Table 14.5 Attitude to deinstitutionalization by the 'unclearness' of the alternative[a]

	Unclearness		
Attitude	Spectators (%)	Bystanders (%)	Participants (%)
Positive	4	4	16
Sceptical	30	36	52
Negative	51	39	30
Hostile	15	21	3
Total	100	100	101
N	159	165	159

Pearson's $r = 0.34$

[a] The attitude variable is a composite measure of the variables shown in Tables 14.1 and 14.2, and the degree of agreement with the following statements: 'I feel secure and informed about what is happening', 'parents will now have to take too large a part in care', 'local authorities are too ignorant about mental retardation to do the job properly'. The variable is collapsed to four categories in the cross-tabulation, but not in the correlation.

PAST INSTITUTIONS AS A FRAME OF REFERENCE

Another obvious reason for parents' opposition could simply be that they were satisfied with the institutional care as it was and saw no reason to change the current form of living. A radical change is always risky, and involves considerable strain, at least in the short run and no one welcomes such strain unless they regard the current situation as dissatisfactory. This is nothing but the logic of Simons' (1945) administrative man: alternative routes of action are considered only if the current situation falls considerably short of ambitions. This section discusses parental satisfaction with the institution, and also the basis for their point of view.

Parents answered several questions on the quality of care and living conditions in present institutions, and the data permit only one conclusion: few other public services would obtain such a positive evaluation from users. Table 14.6 shows the frequency distribution on the question: 'Do you think the institution is providing quality care for your son/daughter?', and nearly 90% express a positive attitude. The same pattern goes for more detailed questions on housing, occupation, leisure, social network, etc. (cf. Tøssebro, 1990b).

Table 14.6 Does the institution, in your opinion, provide quality care to the person to whom you are related?

	%
Yes, high quality	39
Yes, fair quality	48
Tolerably	11
No, poor quality	2
No, very poor quality	0
Total	100
N	452

This means that a service system which is closed down because the living conditions are regarded as disgraceful – by the parents' society, a public committee, the ministry and parliament – is, according to parents, satisfactory. Why this difference? There are probably numerous explanations, but the parents' frame of reference is likely to be involved. When the public committee report recommended dismantling of institutions, this was based on a frame of reference associated with normalization, including living conditions which are decent according to standards applicable to every citizen. The institutions fell considerably short of such standards (cf. Chapter 5).

What about the parents? What is their frame of reference? It is impossible to answer such a question definitely, since the frame of reference is usually tacit and cannot be simply obtained from a postal questionnaire. However, during the telephone calls many parents, without prompting, referred to the past. 'It used to be dreadful, but now it is wonderful' was, in one way or another, repeatedly stated. It was as if the current institutions had saved their child from a tragic past. For example:

> I was crying all the way home the day we left him back at the institution. 'What have I done?' The first years were horrible; 30 of them on the ward – it was pure sadness. Today is different. Now they have a good time there, only six on the ward, and he has got a room of his own. There is even a swimming pool there. It is sad that it is to be closed now, when they have such a good time there.

This story illustrates two things of interest. Firstly, this mother is obviously comparing the present with the past. Secondly, she applies some kind of special frame of reference fit for her mentally retarded son: I assume that she would not have found it so nice for her son to be living six on the ward and with a room of his own if he was a 'normal' 30-year-old son. She expresses a decoupling of a normal frame of reference, and a recoupling to low expectations and past experiences. And in such a perspective, it is reasonable to argue that 'she cannot be better off than now' (another parent's statement).

A different illustration of the same phenomenon is that there were extreme differences in how the same institution was described by parents. To some 'she is having a good time there', to others 'it is unfit as a place to live'. The difference is nearly all explicable by the dummy variable representing the present/past. Those who had their son or daughter living in the institution referred to, described it positively, but if their children had moved to a new place (usually a smaller institution), some time ago or recently, the description was negative. A similar phenomenon is observed by Booth *et al.* (1990).

This interpretation of the qualitative data also draws some support from the association between parental satisfaction and years since institutionalization. Of the parents of those institutionalized prior to 1958 72% are very satisfied, while the corresponding figure for parents of those institutionalized later than 1983 is 47% (Table 14.7 gives variable description). The correlation is weak (0.13), but that is an underestimate. Those

Table 14.7 Attitude to deinstitutionalization by satisfaction with institutions[a]

| | Institutions are | | | |
Attitude	Tolerable (%)	Good (%)	Splendid (%)	Ideal (%)
Positive	17	12	5	0
Sceptical	49	51	34	23
Negative	30	33	44	50
Hostile	5	4	16	27
Total	101	100	99	100
N	66	113	259	44

[a] The satisfaction with institutions variable is composed by 13 variables describing satisfaction with different aspects of the institutional life of the resident – loading 0.54 – 0.81 on the same factor in factor analysis after principal component analysis and varimax rotation. The variable is collapsed to four categories in the cross-tabulation, but not in the correlation.

recently institutionalized are more frequently living in the new, small institutions, and some priority is paid to the younger residents. This means that living conditions are generally better for those recently institutionalized, but their parents are less satisfied – indicating a frame of reference that is not influenced by past institutional care.

The hypothesis that parents of residents in mental retardation institutions in Norway are applying a looking-back frame of reference is obviously in need of a firmer empirical base. However, the numerous telephone calls have convinced me that in order to understand the parents' attitudes, the frame of reference is important.

Frame of reference must not be mixed up with idealizing, though the data also indicates the existence of the latter. For example, parents tend to describe the living conditions as considerably better than staff do, and more important, parents' satisfaction is inversely related to the frequency of contact between parent and resident ($r=0.18$). It is tempting to ask whether the institutions seem better the less you know about them: idealization flourishes when confrontations with reality are rare.

The different frame of reference represents ambitions lower than those of the parental society and the public committee. A socio-political élite preoccupied with normalization and integration obviously regards institutions differently from a group of parents fortunate to be relieved of the misery of past institutions.

To conclude this section Table 14.7 documents the relationship between deinstitutionalization and satisfaction. One-third of those regarding institutions as tolerable or good reject deinstitutionalization, compared with two-thirds among those describing the institutions as splendid and ideal.

In summary, parents' opposition to deinstitutionalization can partly be explained or understood by their satisfaction with the present conditions and this, in turn, is affected by their looking-back frame of reference: a decoupling from current social policy standards. Parents would certainly be happy with incremental improvements, but a revolution is a risky experiment, and contradictory to the logic of satisfying behaviour (Simon, 1945).

This explanation implies a causal order, but this could equally well be the other way around. Favourable attitudes to institutions might be a reaction to the threatening event coming up: dismantling and local responsibility. Anxiousness is very likely to produce defence of the status quo. However, if this was the direction of the causal link, one would expect a substantial correlation between unclearness and satisfaction and statistical interaction between unclearness and satisfaction on opposition to deinstitutionalization. None of this is the case, supporting that causal order is from satisfaction to opposition.

SATISFACTION AND LACK OF CLARITY COMBINED

There are probably many mechanisms affecting parents' attitudes to dein-stitutionalization, both to the specific reform implemented in Norway and to dismantling institutions in general. This chapter is not written with the intention of sorting out all such mechanisms, but to show how oppo-sition can be explained by the vagueness of the alternative and satisfac-tion with contemporary institutions. Regression analysis shows that other variables, such as institution size, attitudes of staff, living conditions, abili-ties of the resident, and parents' characteristics, did not have any impact except sometimes through satisfaction or unclearness. There is one excep-tion to this: parents with low frequency of contact with the resident are more likely to reject deinstitutionalization. The impact is minor, but thought provoking (Table 14.8).

Table 14.9 shows, in percentages, the combined effect of unclearness and satisfaction on opposition. The number of cases are occasionally low but there is no doubt about the general pattern.

Table 14.8 Attitude to deinstitutionalization: multiple regression analysis (r, beta and R^2)

	r	beta	R^2
Alternative 'unclearness'	−0.34	−0.33	
Satisfaction with institutions	0.33	0.32	
Frequency of contact with resident	0.18	0.09	
			0.25

Table 14.9 Percentage of parents negative or hostile to deinstitutionalization by 'unclearness of alternative' and satisfaction with institutions

Unclearness	Satisfaction	Attitude to deinstitutionalization
Participants	tolerable	16*
	good	21
	splendid	39
	ideal	50*
By-standers	tolerable	26
	good	45
	splendid	69
	ideal	87*
Spectators	tolerable	58
	good	49
	splendid	72
	ideal	93*

* = no. of cases less than 20.

CONCLUSION

The picture that emerges is that on the one hand, there is a social policy élite consisting of key persons in the parents' society, a public committee, the ministry and parliament. This alliance evaluates institutions from a frame of reference close to some vague concept of normalization. They are familiar with the ups, downs, delays and practices of local public planning, they are well-informed on what is happening, and their personal risk is low – others must pay the price of failure. On the other hand, the ordinary parent or family has some kind of looking-back frame of reference, they are satisfied with contemporary institutions, the alternative is unclear, they are distant from local planning, and the costs of failure may be considerable. Hence, differences in opinion should not be difficult to understand.

In relation to the parental society, this description sounds very much like an old phenomenon, the iron law of oligarchy (Michels, 1962): the top of an organization in interaction with other élites, while ordinary members are by-passed. In such a situation, a Norwegian sociologist would habitually support the weaker party. The weaker party, however, is not the parents, but the residents.

In this chapter, I have approached parental opposition to institutional closure by trying to understand the parents' reactions, but at the same time disregarding the fact that they may be right. It is necessary to ask the question whether there could be something parents have understood or experienced – something that the parental society, the ministry and myself have failed to see? Let us return to the details on parents' opposition. I argued that it is not accurate to call their attitude a rejection of ideological principles, but rather that they regarded the reform as based on wishful thinking. The key question is the realism of the intended changes in the everyday life of the person with mental retardation. It is obviously not possible to address such a question properly in a closing comment, but I would like to direct attention to the mother claiming that 'the retarded will never be normal'. It is premature to conclude that she has not understood what normalization means. It is as likely that her statement was based on experience – experience of having a non-normal child in a normal society; experiences of stigmatization. Parents, myself included, know that labels like 'citizen' or 'person' are polite, but deceptive. The real world is not that nice, and against such a background, it should be easy to see that talk about integration and normalization may seem – and be – illusory.

On the other hand, the international literature on deinstitutionalization largely presents the new services as better – and, when the lack of clarity is gone, parents' attitudes tend to turn in favour of dismantling. If such documentation were not available, the parents' opposition would not be a puzzle, but plain disagreement.

An earlier version of this paper was previously published in Norwegian: 'Hvorfor saa negative?' i Sandvin (red.): *Mot normalt*, Kommuneforlaget. Oslo, 1992

From complaining to campaigning

15

Hilary Brown, Danuta Orlowska and Jim Mansell

INTRODUCTION

The introduction of new legislation about community care in Britain and increasing financial constraints (Chapter 1) raises many concerns for parents of people with learning disabilities about the level and quality of services available to their sons and daughters. Parents' groups are one vehicle for the expression of such concerns. The ability of such groups to exert pressure on services is one important factor in the development and maintenance of high quality provision for people with learning disabilities. This chapter reports some preliminary work on understanding parents' groups and their role.

Although parents may act alone, Darling (1988, p.152) points out that: 'Parent groups provide an opportunity to learn about effective techniques, to realise that authority can be successfully challenged, and to mobilise for parent action'. However, this optimistic view of groups greatly simplifies the issues involved, as parent groups may serve a variety of functions and interests. Our long-term aim is to find out what it takes to underpin parent organizations so that they can become an effective lobby in the pursuit of community-based, comprehensive services which are tailored to their son or daughter's needs. We are aware that many parents prefer more cautious service options and we are interested to know why, and to explore under what circumstances parents, individually or collectively, feel that they can push back the boundaries and demand something better for their adult children.

At this stage of the work we are beginning to define terms and formulate questions. These are clustered around two pivotal issues: what factors influence parents in what they want for their sons and daughters and how are they to be effective in achieving their aims? We are interested in what triggers parents to shift from accommodating to poor services to campaigning for better ones: in how they go about mobilizing support for change and bringing pressure to bear on decision-makers and politicians. We are interested in the tactics they use, the routes they choose and in what works.

In this chapter we want to review typologies and key issues which emerge from the literature on self-help groups and from our early consultations with national and local parent organizations. One such issue is professionalization and the relationship between parent organizations and the statutory services. We then propose a classification scheme which focuses on action rather than group characteristics because one hypothesis we have at this stage is that organizational aspects of traditional parents' groups may run counter to the achievement of their stated aims, or even jeopardize the emergence of campaigns for quality. Thus instead of form following function we see situations in which form limits function and impedes effective action.

BACKGROUND

Specific action, either to prevent abuse and neglect or to promote choice and quality, takes place against a long history of disagreement about the principles and practice of new service models. Parents' concerns about community-based services have included their instability, structure and layout, safety, expertise of staff and groupings of residents (Frohboese and Sales, 1980). Parents also fear that medical and behavioural needs cannot be met (op. cit.). Issues such as sexual abuse or challenging behaviour confirm parents' fears that the normalization ideology underpinning new service models does not take enough account of the 'differentness' of their sons or daughters.

Despite rhetoric about welcoming complaints, parents who did seek to become involved with their sons and daughters were, and are now, often dissuaded (Frohboese and Sales, op. cit.). When residential services were offered in hospitals, parents were asked to make a clean break by leaving their son or daughter and not visiting for a month (Brown and Bailey, 1986). There was a clear demarcation line between the care being offered by the state and that being offered by the family. More recently community care policies have tended to move away from the practice of usurping parents towards providing specific 'packages' of care to 'prop them up' (Brown and Smith, 1993). Where well-staffed services exclude someone from a service, for example as a result of challenging behaviour or difficult sexual behaviour, parents, irrespective of their wishes or resources, have to pick up the duty to care by default. Thus many parents dread the withdrawal of the scarcely adequate services they currently receive and will not risk upsetting the status quo unless the service has breached very basic standards. Furthermore, competition for scarce resources means that parents may have to present as being unable, rather than unwilling, to cope with caring in order to qualify for a service at all. In doing so they put themselves at further disadvantage in relation to the service provider.

Parents are also concerned about their own needs and those of other members of the family. Brown and Smith (1989) point out that the new service models, framed in terms of choice for individuals who use the service, neglect parents' secondary reliance on services to enable them to work or attend to other family relationships or activities. Because the service is never explicitly acknowledged as being for the parent as well as for their son or daughter, their voices are easily silenced: they can be characterized as neither unbiased advocates for their relatives nor legitimate complainants on their own behalf.

Lack of information about either availability of, or eligibility for, resources, combined with low expectations and few exemplars of what is possible, create a uniquely disempowering dynamic. Parents have come to see the service as a 'help' rather than a 'right'.

This focuses our interest on the conditions which facilitate the alliance of relatively disadvantaged people (in this case parents of people with learning disabilities) and galvanize them into taking action. Left, literally, to their own devices, what constitutes the threshold below which powerless people remain isolated and unable to challenge the resources available to them or their families? If professionals intervene, do they induce, assist or merely subvert the birthing process? It is to the generic self-help literature that we have turned to illuminate these dynamics.

DEFINITION AND ORIGINS

One of the most commonly quoted definitions of self-help groups describes them as:

> Small group structures for mutual aid and the accomplishment of a special purpose ... formed by peers who have come together for mutual assistance in satisfying a common need, overcoming a common handicap or life disrupting problem and bringing about desired social and/or personal change. The initiators and members of such groups perceive that their needs are not, and cannot be, met by or through existing social institutions.
>
> (Katz and Bender, 1976, p.9).

Parent groups are easily encompassed by this definition, although they may sometimes see their needs as being met within the statutory system, (e.g. through schools) and may include members who do not share the common need but support the interests of those who do.

Gartner and Riessman (1977) characterize self-help groups as 'spontaneously' emerging from a 'condition of powerlessness'. Katz and Bender (1976) concur that they are essentially 'voluntary' and emphasize this 'spontaneous origin' as a distinguishing feature. But descriptions which characterize processes as 'spontaneous', 'voluntary' or 'natural' tend to be used naïvely when we are at the limits of our understanding and/or to veil transactions and transformations which involve inequality (Rowbotham, 1973). An alternative hypothesis might be that some self-help groups do not 'emerge' but are manipulated into being, for example to prop up statutory services or to provide services which do not draw on the public purse. Killilea's review (1976) included groups which had originated from more directive involvement of professionals: groups as adjuncts to professionals (as a solution to the shortage of personnel) and as an element in a planned system of care. Levy (1976) also points to the origin of self-help groups as a defining characteristic but includes groups which had been initiated by professionals and subsequently 'go it alone'.

PROBLEM FOCUS

Another common basis on which typologies of self-help groups have been attempted has been their particular 'problem focus' or 'hardship'. Levy's (1976) classification included groups which meet together for personal growth, behaviour control/change, raising status and survival in the face of being labelled deviant. But these categorizations inevitably leak into those which deal with the function of groups, as the way the problem is stated inevitably leads towards certain kinds of solutions. Powell (1987) includes both problem and 'mission' in a five category scheme (Table 15.1).

Parental groups uncomfortably straddle several of these categories. While they may share some of the aims of 'physical handicap' groups in seeking resources their main dichotomy lies in the extent to which the groups are formed to ease the stress of being a carer or to advocate on behalf of their sons and daughters. Clearly the two are not independent of each other, for while better services for people with learning disabilities can often improve the quality of life for their carers there are potential conflicts of interest: increased flexibility and choice for service users can signify less 'reliability' for parents. Increased 'risk taking' and independence for people with learning disabilities can result in more anxiety for their carers.

To what extent does this lack of differentiation hamper parents in

Table 15.1 Problem and mission of parents' organizations[1]

Problem	Mission
habit-disturbance, e.g. addiction	behavioural change
general purpose, e.g. anxiety states, abusive tendencies, loss	various
life style organizations	to overcome discrimination and provide mutual support
significant other organizations	advocate social reform and mutual support for relatives of people with problems
physical handicap	maximize adaptation and provide resources and/or psychological support

[1]Adapted from Powell (1987).

effectively seeking change either on their own behalf or on behalf of their sons and daughters? One hypothesis might be that parents have to couch their own needs in terms of the needs of their sons and daughters and that, in the tradition of Maslow's hierarchy, they dare not advocate for innovative services for their sons and daughters if the provision of them will either compromise basic coping strategies within their own families or involve them significantly in running or managing the improved service. In other words, the crucial question for parents is who is to be 'helped' and on whose shoulders will 'helping' fall?

FUNCTIONS

The most useful dimension to emerge from these typologies is the dichotomy between an internal, member-orientated focus and an external, advocacy and campaigning focus. This we would expect to see reflected in the way problem areas are defined and managed as well as in the activities and constitution of the groups. To what extent do functions cut across each other and what would the optimal balance be? Few groups concentrate exclusively on one function or activity as Richardson and Goodman (1983, p.141) remark of these typologies:

> To the extent that they suggest that individual groups tend to direct themselves to a single purpose only or even primarily, they obscure a proper understanding of the nature of self help groups as a whole ... they can perform a number of functions at the same time.
> (Richardson and Goodman, 1983, p.141)

Lobbying is only one of a range of activities which parent groups undertake. It is one of the five basic functions listed by Richardson and Goodman (1983), the others being: emotional support, the provision of information and advice, direct service provision, social and pressure group activities. In a study of two self-help groups Trojan *et al.* (1990), describe the following functions:

- lobbying: informing the public, organising social action, building coalitions with other initiatives and cooperation with statutory services;
- self-maintenance activities: building consensus, cohesiveness and organising material resources for the group;
- mutual aid activities: sharing experiences, giving mutual information, emotional and practical support, and learning new behaviours if appropriate;
- socialising activities;
- voluntary work: (targeted at non-members) such as advice, advocacy, practical support, empowerment and complementing statutory services.

By placing our emphasis on lobbying we do not wish to downplay the existence or importance of any other function but to explore whether people who have come together for mutual support make good campaigners and conversely what kinds of support campaigners need to optimize their impact on services.

The extent to which parent groups take part in parent action has been addressed at a local branch level by several authors in Britain. Tyne (1978) reported that over half of 24 parent groups were not involved in work on local policy. More recently, a survey of a 50% sample of local groups of a national parents' organization (Mencap, the Royal Society for Mentally Handicapped Children and Adults) (Richardson and Goodman, 1983) was conducted to find out how many were involved in action around issues of local or national policy in the past year. Of responding groups 36% had taken action on two or more issues and 20% on one; 11% were uncertain of how many issues and 34% had not taken any action: actions reported were predominantly at a local level. Of the individual members of the parents' organization surveyed, 27% indicated that they had been involved in campaigning action.

Despite variations in its extent and a certain lack of specificity about what is entailed, parent action is clearly important to members of parent groups. Several researchers have examined the perceived benefits of campaigning to members of parent groups. For example, Bradshaw *et al.*, (1977) found that 42% of parents in their study who were members of voluntary organizations found them to be 'a great help' in 'making the authorities more aware of the problems of families with handicapped children'. More recently, 46% of members of the parents' organization in Richardson and Goodman's study (1983) listed 'working to improve the situation of those with the condition generally' as an important benefit of membership: it emerged as the highest rated benefit of eight, and Ayer and Alaszewski (1984) reported that 60% of mothers of children with special needs who belonged to voluntary associations thought they were a 'great help' in 'campaigning for improvement in services'. From these studies, it is clear that the lobbying focus is an important one to some members, although parents no doubt join for different reasons and have different priorities for their involvement.

REPRESENTATIVENESS OF MEMBERS AND LEADERS

Research on self-help groups has suggested that members of self-help groups tend not to be representative of the general population. In a review of studies about help-seeking behaviour, Gourash (1978) [cited by Katz (1981)] notes that young, white, educated and middle-class women seek assistance both from self-help groups and professionals more than males, minorities, older people, people with less than high school education and the lower- and working-classes. Katz (1961) argued that horizontal communication between members distinguished them from conventional social agencies and Balgopal *et al.* (1986) generalize that self-help groups typically reflect equal status among members with hierarchies existing purely for organizational and operational purposes. However, given that groups are part of a wider social environment, and one in which inequality is endemic, we hypothesize that differences in status on account of gender, race and age are bound to be salient within parent groups and affect the processes that occur.

There is evidence to back up this view in that membership of parent groups seems not to be representative. In a survey of four local branches of the American Association for Retarded Citizens, Segal (1969) found that the proportion of parents who joined varied from 30%–92%. Both parent and non-parent members were almost exclusively white, mostly women, of higher socioeconomic status and generally older. His discussion with informants suggested the operation of racial discrimination when black people participated which discouraged their involvement. The lack of younger people was attributed to such parents being more willing to fight for services directly and tending to join groups affiliated to the school system.

More recently, in a survey of members of a national parents' organization in Britain, Richardson and Goodman (1983) found that 76% were current parents, 3% former parents and 20% other supporters. Race and gender were not explored, but higher socioeconomic status was evident with 40% from professional or intermediate status households, 38% skilled and 16% semi-skilled or unskilled. With regard to age, 60% of members were 50 years old or over.

These figures suggest that groups may not be representative of parents of people with learning disabilities, particularly given the association of mild learning disabilities with socioeconomic disadvantage. There is particular concern about the low levels of participation of parents from ethnic minority communities leading to professional initiatives to set up groups with these parents in mind. Furthermore where parents from lower status groups do join their issues may not be taken up.

The leaders of self-help groups may also be unrepresentative of potential or actual members. Schubert and Borkman (1991) offered a range of mechanisms for the choice of leaders including:

- any member being able to volunteer for leadership;
- members being trained for leadership positions;
- the provision of trained and possibly paid leaders;
- professionals deciding the selection and roles of leaders.

Segal's (1969) study of the American Association of Retarded Citizens, found that 72% of parent and non-parent respondents wanted the director to be a paid professional: and in fact most state level executive directors were white, male, married, had a college or graduate school education, previous experience in health, welfare, education or business and were not parents of children with learning disabilities. However, less is known about leaders at local level.

Clearly the dynamics of parent action and the emergence of themes around which action is focused are complicated by many factors including social inequality. Many parents do not belong to parent groups and although parent action is seen as important by many members, it is not an activity carried out by all groups. Where the group does take action, not all parents are involved and the issues selected for campaigning may not equally reflect the concerns of all members. At each stage of this filter, therefore, various realms of parental concern are in danger of being overlooked in the parent action process: as Richardson and Goodman (1983, p. 141) point out: ' ... people with a "common" condition may not, in fact, be addressing themselves to the same basic problems at all'. Hence the emergence of particular issues is an important area to examine: whose interests are being met by action and who is doing the acting?

RELATIONSHIPS WITH EXTERNAL AGENCIES AND PROFESSIONALS

The question of the involvement of professionals is 'one of the most often discussed, crucial, and vexing posed by the reemergence of self-help groups' (Katz, 1981, p.145). Kurtz (1990) has argued that cooperation with professionals is important because professionals can then refer potential members to the group and because self-help groups benefit from the support and credibility of professionals. However, if as Richardson and Goodman (1983, p.143) point out: 'Many self-help groups consider the benefits or services provided by statutory authorities to their members to be inadequate, and therefore take some measures to bring about change', the involvement of professionals who work for those same statutory authorities may make the definition of the issues they are fighting for more difficult (e.g. Kalifon, 1991).

The critical issue is the extent to which parent organizations are infiltrated by and/or dependent on professionals and service agencies, and whether 'consumer-owned' groups can usefully be delineated from 'professionally-owned' groups. In developing a typology Schubert and Borkman (1991) explore the relationship between self-help groups and external agencies, such as funding bodies, statutory service providers, national voluntary agencies, and the involvement of professionals inside the group as initiators, members, workers, decision-makers, or other key players.

There is clearly a continuum from autonomous self-help groups which exist independently, and can thereby risk criticizing services, to 'client' self-help groups, set up and maintained by professional agencies as a facet of service provision rather than an independent voice. Schubert and Borkman (op. cit.) review the 'resource dependence perspective' formulated by Gross and Etzioni (1985) which postulates that:

> To the extent an organisation received resources from some external source, [it]... became resource dependent upon that source, thereby giving up some autonomy over its own functioning.
>
> (Gross and Etzioni, 1985)

They cite Pfeffer (1981, p.106) who proposes that a 10% stake is enough to give the funding body considerable control.

However, access to, as well as dependence on, other agencies is a key factor in campaigning activities and may seem to provide an important 'trade-off'. For example, parent representatives have generally been accepted as participants within the planning process, albeit within a 'token' framework, i.e. those concerned may have neither capacity, roles or networks which enable them to exercise real power (Drake, 1992). The extent to which, either individual parent representatives or parent groups as a whole have the potential to influence the processes of statutory agencies and purchasing authorities is open to question.

An examination of the role of professionals within groups reveals the extent to which parent groups and professional workers are intertwined and demonstrates the pervasive dynamic of professionalization within such groups. Katz (1961) proposed a 'natural history' or cycle in parent groups from the group's origins in informal organization, to the emergence of leadership, formal organization and ultimately professionalization, but he later (Katz and Bender, 1976) highlighted self-help groups which resist professionalization. In Schubert and Borkman's (1991) typology, professionals are seen to have varying amounts of influence, from none, through various advisory roles to leadership and control. Although Back and Taylor (1976) mention that distrust of professionals is a striking characteristic of adherents of self-help, the growth of groups from small-scale one-off structures to national and even international organizations is inevitably accompanied by the increased use of professional workers at all levels to fulfil functions which members themselves dealt with in the initial stages.

The move from an amateur to a professionally-run organization is sometimes hailed as a victory for progressive attitudes but it can toll the death knell for effective parent power as they lose the necessary power and resources to enable them to provide a service of their choice. Agencies thereby lose their distinctive nature as parent-led and instead take their place as mainstream providers of services. These agencies cannot be presented as independent of government at either a national or local level, they are more in the position of 'client' states than independent territories and, having been well and truly colonized, are inevitably compromised in providing feedback to their paymasters. Schubert and Borkman (op. cit.) combine these two dimensions (external and internal dependence on professionals) to produce a typology of groups ranging from unaffiliated to federated, affiliated to hybrid and finally to managed groups.

Interaction with and assistance from professionals is clearly an important issue. Appropriate levels of professional involvement have been considered to be those which are responsive to the needs of the group (e.g. Balgopal, Ephross and Vassil, 1986) and to be optimum when there is neither over-involvement nor under-involvement (Kurtz, 1990) – a fine balance for both groups and professionals to strike. If parents are to campaign effectively what kind of support, information and resources do they need from professional workers and statutory agencies? What is the balance between parents being served by professionals and being enlisted in campaigns which have their origins in professional self-interest?

PARENT ACTION AS THE KEY CLASSIFICATION VARIABLE

Each of the typologies discussed highlights useful dimensions against which parent groups in their many guises can be categorized. A development of our thinking occurred when we began to categorize the action itself rather than group characteristics. In creating this focus, we wanted to encapsulate a range of actions which parents, as individuals, in groups or as parties to wider alliances, could take to challenge the services available to them and their sons and daughters. What is clarified in this framework is the relationship between action and existing service provision.

We have created a matrix of activities from complaining to campaigning in which parents or parent groups can get involved, sometimes in support of radical service options over mainstream service provision and sometimes working against professional 'enlightenment'. By focusing on the relationship of the group to mainstream services it is possible to make links between the organizational and functional aspects of groups which oppose, resist, support, challenge and break away from the mainstream. The continuum of activity which we propose classifies the aim of the activity in relation to current services and moves from activities we describe as preventing, improving, maintaining, extending, augmenting or replacing current service provision.

The continuum works independently of the kinds of services parents want. For example, at one end of the continuum parents may step in to prevent bad practice but they may also block a radical programme of sex education or of self-advocacy. At the other end, parents may forego services in favour of innovative and individualized models or they may opt out to seek more institutionalized service provision if they do not trust the community-based options on offer. In Figure 15.1 we give examples which demonstrate the actions of parents active in seeking community-based service options for their sons or daughters: however, this model could also have been documented in relation to parental opposition to deinstitutionalization and empowering models of care.

This span of actions can be undertaken on behalf of individuals or of groups, and by individual parents or groups. National parent organizations may also grow up around these separate functions as well as around the specific issues they select as the foci of their campaigns.

In supporting parents seeking positive service options using this model we can look at the risks and potential benefits of different strategies. At each end of the continuum, where parents are either complaining about

Aim in relation to existing service	Prevent	Improve	Maintain	Extend	Augment	Replace
Definition	Here the aim is to close a bad service or remove an individual member of staff. Examples include ward closure, exposing abuse, mismanagement or severe limitations in quality	In this case the aim is to change one aspect of the service without jeopardizing other aspects, this will usually take the form of a complaint or campaign *against* a particular aspect of practice	Here the goal is to protect the service from threatened cut-backs or contraction – the concern is to maintain availability and not allow standards to slip	Expanding the service and gaining access for additional service users adds up to a 'more of the same' approach wherein quantity and access to the service will be a more important issue than quality	Here the emphasis is to add on a new component to an existing service or programme meeting additional or specialized needs without removing the current core activities. In this case there will be a campaign *for* something new to be added to the service	In this mode parents will create an innovative service and be willing to let go of an existing service in order to create a new model over which they can exercise some control in the planning phase, possibly throughout implementation and almost certainly in ongoing quality control
Example at an individual level	Challenging physical or sexual abuse of an individual through the courts	Complaining about lack of leisure activities in a group home for an individual with multiple handicaps	Refusing to allow an individual's day placement to be reduced from five days a week to three	Asking for respite care every fortnight rather than once a month	Campaigning for access to a generic mental health service for someone with a learning disability and an additional mental health problem	Using the care management process to plan an alternative day service for an individual with special needs to replace segregated provision with supported, community-based activities

Example at local group level	Closure of a ward, hostel or deregistration of a private home after ongoing abuse has been discovered	Campaigning for improved staffing ratios at the weekend so that residents of a group home are able to go out and participate in household activities	Lobbying councillors to prevent charges for day services currently provided free of charge and to prevent reduction in the service county-wide	Campaigning for more group homes so that people currently living with their families do not have a worse service than people moving out of hospital	Campaigning for speech therapy services in an area to meet the needs of children assessed under the 1981 Education Act	Designing and setting up a parent led supported employment service which enabled people with learning disabilities to come off benefits
Example at national or policy level	Campaigning to stop institutional provision	Redirection of resources to improve quality of residential environments	Public campaign to oppose cuts in services	Campaign to increase national availability of day places	Use of legislation and legal precedents to establish rights to speech therapy for all children under the 1981 Education Act	National policy framework to establish innovative services for people with challenging behaviours

Figure 15.1 Continuum of parent action where parents seek more radical alternatives to statutory provision.

major issues or campaigning for services to meet significant unmet needs, they come nearer to putting their current level of service in jeopardy. This they will do only if they perceive themselves both as having nothing to lose and as being able to cope if the current service is withdrawn. It may take extremes to reach this point, for example, where a service is so damaging that they feel they cannot allow it to continue or where they are so inspired by the advantages of new models that they are willing to give up a secure but unsatisfactory option. Going for quality is made more likely where parents have some 'bridge' back to a stable service if innovation falters.

SUPPORTING PARENT ACTION

Another purpose of working within a framework which is built around the impact of parent action is that it suggests the kind of information and support which might facilitate successful outcomes in each category of action. The resources a group has – both latent and manifest in terms of the skills and contacts of its members, past history of parent action and relationships with other bodies – may affect the tactics and route a parent group takes. Local groups can act on their own, with the advice of their national organization if they have one, or turn to a consortium of bodies or umbrella organization for advice. But the continuum also suggests that different kinds of action may require different strategies and that these need to be reflected in group structure and organization. To be successful each kind of campaign may emerge out of, and draw on the resources of, a different kind and size of group.

Preventing specific practices is most likely to be achieved by small groups of parents whose adult sons and daughters use the same service and who may need to ally themselves with professionals, who are willing to be whistle-blowers, for mutual protection and credibility. They are likely to need legal input and knowledge of formal complaint systems. Seeking to improve existing provision is more likely to be successful if the group are involved in ongoing monitoring and feedback. A standing parent committee, for example, which develops good relationships with management will be able to draw on these links in demanding better quality without formalizing complaints or putting the continuity of the service in jeopardy.

Resisting closure and cutbacks (maintaining and extending services) is part of a more visible political lobby where mass membership is necessary to mobilize a campaign through mainstream political channels. Letter-writing, picketing council meetings and using the local and national media are likely to be important tactics. Extending services also relies on a groundswell to create public awareness of shortfalls.

Campaigning to augment specific services is likely to be undertaken by a smaller group of parents united by the fact that their sons and daughters share a particular disability and that they share a particular view about what is an appropriate service for them. Networking will initially be important if parents in the same situation are to find each other and work on common issues. Specialist knowledge may be required if a group are seeking services which address specific disabilities or aspire to innovative intervention and treatment.

Thus action at both ends of the continuum demands a small group of highly committed people, who are likely to share a similar philosophy, and have sons and daughters at a similar stage of development. Common needs, such as the need for future residential services, or respite care, may crystallize around transitions such as the move from school to adult services, institutional closure, or the fear of older parents about what will happen to their children when they are no longer able to care for them. Timescale is important. Also important is the extent to which 'opters out' have to be willing to invest time in the long-term running of the service they have planned. If they hand it over to professional agencies their model can be corrupted unless organizational mechanisms are put in place to facilitate ongoing parental control and monitoring. On the other hand, models of innovative professionally-run services also need to be made available so that in demanding replacement services of high quality, parents do not have to place themselves outside the boundaries of public-sector provision. Meanwhile professionals who urge parents to seek quality services for their sons and daughters should acknowledge that as long as innovation is perceived as a 'do-it-yourself' model it may prove too expensive in terms of input as well as too risky in terms of output.

Conversely large, loose-knit local groups are better suited to campaigns which maintain/extend existing service provision than to campaigns which innovate or advocate for specialized programmes. Amorphous groups, such as those local branches of national parents' organizations which grow up around day-centres or hospital closure, tend towards the 'no change' or the 'more of the same' models and we can conceptualize these mid-points as a kind of 'bulge'. Deriving like-minded, clearly focused groups from such organizations through targeted networking might be a prerequisite for more effective lobbying, a kind of service 'matchmaking' to ensure that parents whose children have similar needs, and who have themselves a similar outlook on service options can meet to pool their resources. Organization of groups on geographical rather than functional criteria is likely to perpetuate a pull towards the status quo.

CONCLUSION

Parents generally have a long-term commitment to the welfare of their sons and daughters with learning disabilities but they are in a vulnerable position when it comes to challenging the services which are on offer. When resources are scarce, parents are inevitably afraid to lose what little they have and are more likely to campaign for incremental change than to risk a complete break either through exposing abuse or transcending mediocrity. Supporting different forms of parent action and organization is an important step in creating checks and balances within the new mixed market of care. While most parents will be struggling to maintain access and coverage, some will aspire towards excellence and others will risk whatever it takes to protect their sons and daughters in the face of unprincipled practice. It is also important to note that successful parent action can work against innovative community-based services as well as providing a momentum for quality. We believe it is important for research to clarify what it will take to create new alliances between parents and professionals, to create new networks within the legal and other advocacy agencies which support parent action, and to work in a way which recognizes and respects the dual role of parents who function both as advocates for their sons and daughters and as carers with legitimate needs and rights of their own.

Conclusion: integrating diverse experience 16

Jim Mansell and Kent Ericsson

INTRODUCTION

This chapter attempts to draw together the themes emerging from the different contributions made earlier, in order both to try to understand what has happened and to identify some of the questions which remain unanswered. At first sight, the deinstitutionalization process in Scandinavia, the United States and Britain appears to spring from different sources at different times, and to have been implemented with different degrees of success. And yet by the mid-1990s there seems to be convergence in the implementation process and at least some of the problems emerging in different countries appear to be the same.

The first part of this chapter addresses the question of what drives the process of deinstitutionalization. Many people working in services for people with intellectual disabilities identify ideological commitment as the primary driving force. They would argue that the energy for change came from the idea of normalization, first in Scandinavia, then in the United States and Britain. But as several contributors note, the course and pace of deinstitutionalization have also depended on other factors of a much more practical nature (like financial incentives) and on other ideological pressures (such as the radical Conservative critique of the welfare state). Despite the variation in timing and acceptance of new philosophies of care, implementation (especially in terms of institutional closure) has occurred at roughly the same time. It is important to try to understand what is the engine driving deinstitutionalization because much remains to be achieved, both in terms of numbers of people still cared for in institutions (in the countries represented in this volume but also in the rest of the world) and in terms of the quality and competence of community services. An appreciation of the interplay of different factors is required in order to sustain, extend and improve the process.

The second part of the chapter attempts to take stock of what has been achieved through the deinstitutionalization process. It is clear from earlier chapters that there are questions to be answered about the impact of institutional closure and the provision of community services on the lives of service users, their families and the staff who provide support to them. It is also appropriate to consider what has been the impact of deinstitutionalization on the service organizations involved in implementing the new policy and on the social policy framework within the countries involved. Deinstitutionalization is probably the major change in services for people needing substantial extra support (intellectual disabilities, mental health needs, old age) in the three geographical areas covered by this book in the last 25 years; how has it changed government and wider social perspectives on the needs of service users and their place in society?

Finally, where does deinstitutionalization now lead? Perhaps the process is drawing to a close as the old institutions are replaced, so that people with intellectual disabilities become ordinary citizens whose needs are largely met through services available to the general population. On the other hand, institutions have been a remarkably durable and resilient form of social organization and there must be at least the possibility that the new services in the community come to recreate institutional practices. Where institutional practices re-emerge the question arises whether this is essentially a technical problem of poor organization and inadequate staff training (as Mansell and Felce imply), or whether it can only be addressed through further reform of the community service model (as Ericsson and Allard imply).

WHAT DRIVES THE PROCESS OF DEINSTITUTIONALIZATION?

As Kent Ericsson shows in relation to Sweden in Chapter 6, the idea of normalization has its roots in the creation of the welfare state at the end of the Second World War, as an expression of an ideological principle of inclusiveness in society. At first, both in Sweden and Norway, new policy was framed in terms of combining better material conditions in institutions for people with severe intellectual disabilities while providing services in the community for people with mild intellectual disabilities. Services were specialized, and both institutions and community services were controlled by central and regional government rather than by local municipalities. National parents' organizations have been partners with government in shaping policy and have been closely identified with the deinstitutionalization movement.

In both countries there has been a high degree of political and social consensus about public services and the general style of policy implementation has been of sustained change over many years, with intermittent review and legislation extending the policy to more severely disabled people on the basis of proven success and satisfaction. The latest stage in this process (from 1985 in Sweden and 1988 in Norway) has been the reintegration of services for people with intellectual disabilities into the local municipal level of government, and the dismantling of the specialist regional tier of organization.

With this has come the final stage of institutional closure, including the replacement of quite small, modernized, expensive institutions. Whereas the dominant model of community residential service in the 1980s was a staffed group home, the newest services are intended to be private apartments with access to some shared facilities and staff support organized on a personal basis. These are relatively expensive services (compared to group homes or institutions), and they are justified principally through the political commitment to providing conditions of life of the same standard for everyone, whether or not people have intellectual disabilities.

In the United States, Braddock *et al.* (1995) has shown that the civil rights of individuals with intellectual disabilities was also the starting point for change. Very poor conditions in institutions were used by parents, often in league with senior staff in intellectual disability services, to challenge the legality initially of the standard of care and then throughout the 1970s to secure the replacement of institutions with community services. Wolfensberger's (1972) reformulation of the principle of normalization around a Lemertian social deviance perspective provided a theoretical framework more suitable for the highly individually focused societies of North America. This approach to normalization probably had more influence in shaping the form of community services rather than in underpinning the decision to close institutions in the first place.

There is much more evidence of conflict in the American experience, with institutions actively defending themselves and only reluctantly being dragged into closure programmes. Parents and the deinstitutionalization lobby have, as Castellani notes in Chapter 3, successfully used the law to more closely define the interpretation of the United States Constitution in this area, eventually (in the Pennhurst case) obtaining a decision that institutional care itself was unconstitutional. This essentially local action has been more important than policy-making at national level, although as Castellani shows in relation to New York State's experience, national funding created important incentives for the development of community services. Some of these incentives were not primarily concerned with intellectual disability issues, such as the way careful checking

244 Conclusion: integrating diverse experience

of standards in an attempt to rein in Medicaid expenditure created incentives to abandon institutions which had been designated as 'intermediate care facilities'.

As in Scandinavia, services for people with intellectual disabilities in the United States have been rather specialized, so that at state level the Office of Mental Retardation (sometimes linked with mental health services) has provided a high level of expertise and commitment. Most of the services provided to replace institutions have been private services (including those provided by not-for-profit agencies) and the same shift from larger (8–10 person 'intermediate care facilities') to smaller service models (3 or 4 people sharing a house) has been evident. Allard (Chapter 7) describes the latest stage in this process, the creation of a new service model ('supported living') intended to more fully achieve ordinary citizenship for people with intellectual disabilities.

In Britain, in contrast to the Scandinavian countries and the United States, formal statements of individual rights are largely absent from the constitution. The deinstitutionalization movement in Britain has been the product of several factors present in the other countries, but not codified nor reinforced by reference to an over-arching legal and political framework. The British deinstitutionalization movement also differs from Scandinavian and American experience in that national parents' groups appear to have played a much less important role in promoting institutional closure, so that it has been a largely professionally- and managerially-led enterprise.

Faced with apparently high demand for residential care and considerable overcrowding British policy, as early as the mid-1950s, attempted to limit the provision of places in institutions to severely disabled people (those 'in need of continuous medical and nursing care'). What happened from then on was that, again and again, researchers and reformers showed that community-based services achieved better results for people at the time falling on the institutional side of this administrative boundary. Service models were influenced by Scandinavian and American experience, but also by the upswelling of academic interest in institutional regimes, especially for children, after the Second World War.

Although this process was given an added stimulus at the end of the 1960s by major scandals in institutions, it was not until the 1980s that large-scale deinstitutionalization was achieved for people with severe intellectual disabilities. As in Sweden and Norway, this started mainly as a change in central government services (the National Health Service) but later reforms gave responsibility for community services to local government. Part of this change was also to adopt a version of the American model of public administration, in which the public authority purchases care mainly from private providers.

Despite many differences between policy and services in Scandinavia, the United States and Britain, deinstitutionalization for people of all levels of disability and the closure of institutions really only started on a large scale in the 1980s: but why was this? Two common features are apparent in the accounts presented here: pressure on institutional costs and the availability of mature models. In broad terms, it seems likely that decisions about resource allocation came to the fore in this period, and that they interacted with evidence of feasibility of the policy and practice of community services. This is not to deny the importance of ideology or philosophy and the wider social acceptance of people with intellectual disabilities as full citizens in their societies; but one has to explain why Sweden and Norway, with long socio-democratic traditions and large public-sector provision should deinstitutionalize at the same time as Britain and the United States who have Conservative governments, bent on dismantling public services and promoting a highly individualistic ideology.

The Scandinavian countries already had a strong commitment to improving living conditions for people with intellectual disabilities; for them, the cost of improving existing institutions – often built since the Second World War – to match the standard of community services would have been prohibitive. In the United States too, the cost of institutional improvement presented decision-makers with a problem: no matter how much resources in institutions were increased, courts most often took the view that they failed their clients. In both these situations, the selection of community-based service options was apparently at least cost-neutral to decision-makers (e.g. Heal, 1987). Actually, as Shumway points out in Chapter 2, in at least some American services, the lower cost of community residential services permitted increases in the number of people served.

The process in Britain seems to have been different, but with the same result. British institutional costs have always been lower than the cost of small services in the community (e.g. Felce, 1993; Cambridge et al., 1994), mainly because increases in institutional costs did not keep pace with funding levels in the other countries. No legal or policy framework existed to drive up institutional costs once barely tolerable standards of care (i.e. not causing scandals) had been achieved. The incoming Conservative Government of 1979 made sustained attempts to reduce public expenditure and, after 1982, reorganized management in the National Health Service along more commercial lines. It seems probable that these new managers took the opportunity to reduce their expenditure by developing community services which utilized social security funding (achieving some cost-shunting as well as increases in staffing levels), closing institutions and realizing the value of large institutional estates (e.g. Audit Commission, 1987). Thus, deinstitutionalization in Britain was also cost-neutral (at least) to the public agencies which provided the institutions. It is this which explains another characteristic of the British situation – the extent to which the process was driven by closure rather than, as elsewhere, by development of community services.

The second contributing factor was the availability of mature models and rationales. During the 1970s the pioneers of community services had demonstrated new service models (typically the staffed group home for a small number of service users). Whereas institutional refurbishment had limited results, these new models were seen as clearly better than the institutions they replaced. Although the first community services focused on people with mild or moderate intellectual disabilities, they now demonstrated their effectiveness and feasibility for people with all levels of intellectual disability. Thus, for example, the Pennhurst case in the United States (Laski, 1980), the publication in Britain of the report *An Ordinary Life* by the influential King's Fund Centre (1980) and the Report of the Committee on Handicap Services (1981) in Sweden all marked the definition of community services as achievable and desirable in the eyes of decision-makers in intellectual disability services.

Just as important as the actual models or forms of services was the availability of administrative mechanisms and procedures which allowed the development of community services. Examples of this include the intermediate care facility funding programme in the United States and the availability of 'dowry' monies for people leaving institutions in Britain and also a much wider group of administrative procedures concerned, for example, with space standards, fire precautions, staffing and personnel practices and control over service users' lives. Whereas the first community services often had to work against prevailing approaches – achieving change in spite of these mechanisms – by the beginning of the 1980s people trying to develop community services had relatively tried and tested methods available to them. By and large, the extension of community services to serve people with severe or profound intellectual disabilities, and the pursuit of institutional closure, was within the competence of administrators and managers to decide: it did not require nor excite great political interest. Indeed, in the United States and in Britain the change was consistent with wider government policies of reducing the scale of the public sector.

It should also be recognized that much of the impetus for reform came from staff within institutional services, who saw new opportunities for meeting the needs of the people they served and for themselves in better services in the community.

Finally, the general social climate concerning disability should not be overlooked. Recognizing the citizenship of people with intellectual disabilities was consistent with a broader social movement: from the civil rights movement to the Americans with Disabilities Act in the United States, race relations, equal opportunities and current attempts to achieve disability rights legislation in Britain, and the development of integrated schooling and a general framework of inclusive civil rights in Sweden.

To summarize this argument, then: the growth and rapid implementation of policies of deinstitutionalization in Scandinavia, the United States and Britain in the 1980s reflects both the development of alternative models of care and the potential costs of effectively humanizing institutions. The supporting ideologies constructed to defend and promote deinstitutionalization were consistent with wider government and social agendas. In Scandinavia, normalization meant the extension of social solidarity to everyone in a welfare state in which a main function of government was to provide for all its people. In the United States, normalization became an individualistic philosophy in which the function of community services was to promote valued individual roles which transgressed group stereotypes, in line with the tradition of promoting individual rights against 'big government'. In Britain, deinstitutionalization was defended on the pragmatic grounds of being better than institutional care, but it was also consistent with 'Thatcherism' and the privatization of care (both in the sense of using private-sector service providers and of expecting families to bear more of the burden and cost of care). In Britain, Sweden and Norway, deinstitutionalization also became consistent with policies of decentralization to local authorities.

WHAT HAVE BEEN THE RESULTS OF DEINSTITUTIONALIZATION?

There can be no doubt that, in general, people with intellectual disabilities have benefited from deinstitutionalization. The appalling conditions that did exist in institutions in Britain and the United States are almost gone, and the institutions are in terminal decline. The mass media look now to Eastern Europe for cruelty and neglect, where once they found them at home. In Norway and Sweden too, the living conditions in community services are better than the relatively new, highly staffed institutions in these countries.

As a number of contributors to this volume have noted, the empirical evidence available suggests that the opportunities provided by better conditions have been translated into better quality of life. In general, people have more normal patterns and rhythms of life; they grow and develop as individuals; they use services and facilities available to the wider community; and they and their relatives express satisfaction. However, as Emerson and Hatton (Chapter 11) show in the British context, this general picture conceals considerable variation for individuals. Institutional practices and outcomes persist or recur in some of the new community services. Clearly this is also true in American services, hence papers with titles like 'Preventing institutionalization in the community' (Landesman, 1988), although the overwhelming picture presented by published research is favourable. In Sweden and Norway the staffed group home has been the subject of continuing criticism for its essentially institutional nature and the drive is to create services around individuals in their own housing.

In Sweden and Norway, improvement in conditions for people with intellectual disabilities appears to have been achieved without disadvantaging families and staff. The right to housing has enabled people with intellectual disabilities to leave home when they and their families wish, and staff from institutions have had the opportunity to work in community services with comparable or better conditions of service. In the United States, too, there has been an overall expansion of residential care (from just over 290 000 in 1977 to nearly 347 000 in 1992 (Braddock *et al.*, 1995)), so that some people with intellectual disabilities formerly required to live with their families because there were insufficient residential services have benefited. For staff in American community services, however, deinstitutionalization has brought poorer conditions of service than staff in the institutions, with instances of people being paid at minimum wage levels (Braddock and Mitchell, 1992). In Britain, there was a net gain in residential places by the mid-1980s (from 56 400 to 59 000 (Audit Commission, 1986)) but more recently there has been evidence of a net loss of about 5000 places as institutional closure accelerates and of an increased burden of care on families (Farmer *et al.*, 1991); it is also the case that the workforce in community services is less well-qualified and less well-paid than in institutions. In both Britain and the United States the picture is, however, very diverse, with good and bad practice coexisting, depending on local circumstances.

Several different but related explanations have been suggested for the continuation or re-emergence of institutional care practices in community services. First, it has been suggested (Mansell *et al.*, 1993) that the implementation process becomes bureaucratic and proceduralized; that the original visionaries move on leaving others (perhaps with less energy, commitment and skill) to produce the large numbers of services actually needed to fulfil the plan. This is a standard problem of policy implementation and deinstitutionalization shows many factors which might lead to it: long timescales, multiple agencies and constituencies, and transfers of responsibility across organizational boundaries. Typical responses to this problem are attempts at greater control by innovators through franchising the original model or at disseminating principles and ideas rather than solutions.

Felce (Chapter 8) and Mansell *et al.* (1993) have suggested that institutional care practices in community services may reflect the failure of planners and managers to understand the relationship between quality of service user lifestyle, patterns of staff performance and management and organization of the service. Decision-makers therefore focus on too limited a set of issues (e.g. concern about buildings and locations) and, when they have achieved what they want in these areas they neglect to follow-through on other, less immediately obvious issues. This relates to the implementation problem described above in that efforts to disseminate models of new services may overlook or fail to emphasize all the components known to be important.

Many contributors to this book have suggested that problems expressed at procedural levels may be linked to ideological problems. Mansell (Chapter 4) suggests that, in the British context, decision-makers may not be particularly committed to improving services above a tolerable level, and that this may help explain why it is so difficult to get managers and staff to focus on the important issues. Tøssebro (Chapter 5) and Sandvin (Chapter 12) both caution against expecting too much to change in services when the way people with intellectual disabilities are seen in society, and the kind of society it is, have not changed.

In relation to this issue Sandvin's observation that one of the processes at work is 'dedifferentiation' is particularly relevant. A major claim of the deinstitutionalization movement has been that people with intellectual disabilities would get better treatment if they had access to the ordinary resources available to other members of society: institutions represented inferior treatment in all sorts of respects. It is clear, however, that a significant proportion of people with intellectual disabilities need help to obtain sufficient access to ordinary resources. For example, some people with intellectual disabilities need staff to help them shop, or go to the theatre, or manage their finances; ordinary community dental or medical services, casualty wards or emergency rooms are often not organized so that people with intellectual disabilities find them usable. If re-entry into the mainstream of society means providing whatever special help is needed to ensure equal access to social goods (as Ericsson suggests the 'citizen perspective' implies in Chapter 6), then dedifferentiation has to avoid special needs becoming invisible.

In concluding this discussion of the effects of deinstitutionalization it is also important to note the effects on service organizations and the wider social policy climate. In all the countries involved, deinstitutionalization has been a developing process in which success at each stage has led people on to more imaginative forms of service (from group homes to supported living, from day activity centres to supported employment). New lives in the community have created new perspectives about what it might be possible to achieve. As Conroy and Feinstein (1990a) and Mansell (1994) note, the frame of reference in the policy debate has shifted away from questioning the feasibility of community services to, on the one hand, technical issues of implementation and on the other, political questions on the desirability of properly meeting people's needs.

WHERE DOES THE MOVEMENT FOR DEINSTITUTIONALIZATION NOW LEAD?

What of the future? Two broad questions need to be addressed: will the process of deinstitutionalization continue, leading to the complete abandonment of institutions as a form of residential care for people with intellectual disabilities, and will people with intellectual disabilities, their families and the staff who support them, experience a better life in community services?

If it is recognized that the process of deinstitutionalization has been driven by factors other than an ideological commitment to better services, then it may be prudent to consider how these factors might change and what impact this might have on the replacement of institutions. It was argued in the first part of this chapter that the pace of deinstitutionalization was sustained in the 1980s because community services cost no more (to the people making the decisions) than institutional care. In Scandinavia and the United States this was largely because of the high cost of institutions but in Britain and the United States it was also due to the opportunity to gain access to new central government funds through community services.

There is evidence in both Britain and the United States that central government concern at the growth of these new areas of expenditure is leading to greater restrictions on their use. In Britain, the use of social security to fund residential care in the community was severely curtailed by new legislation at the end of the 1980s, largely in response to substantial increases in the number of elderly people entering private nursing homes, and under the new arrangements local authority social services departments are expected to fund all residential care costs. In the United States, Castellani (Chapter 3) shows how in New York there has been increasing pressure through certification procedures to restrict access to federal funding.

These pressures create incentives in two directions. First, planners can reduce costs by reverting to larger services with lower staffing ratios, i.e. they can return to institutional models of care. Alternatively, they can redefine very small-scale residential care – supported living – as a form of domiciliary service so that the individual continues to be entitled to social security funding. As Mansell (Chapter 4) and Braddock *et al.* (1995) report, there are larger private-sector residential homes in Britain and the United States and these appear to be relatively untouched by the ideology of deinstitutionalization. The institutional legacy may therefore live on and may be capable of expansion if policies change. Clearly there is also the development of supported living and it may be that these two trends will continue to coexist in future in the absence of clear national policies about service models.

Two other policy influences seem likely to bear upon the further progress of deinstitutionalization. The first is the perceived success and value of community care. The commitment in principle to deinstitutionalization was often formed before people had much experience of community services: as Sandvin (Chapter 12) notes, it was as much a reaction to conditions in institutions as a positive vision of future possibilities. Once community services exist, their benefits (for people with intellectual disabilities, but also for service organizations and governments) can be more readily assessed. If in fact community services are not very good, or too much trouble, then a lobby for recreating institutional care may emerge. This has happened in Britain (an organization called Rescare) and in the United States there have recently been comments from influential politicians about the attractiveness of inexpensive congregate care (Croser, 1995). There is therefore a need to address the problems of quality of community services raised by several contributors to this volume, to continue to amass data on the various benefits of good services and how these compare with others (for example, in the way that Conroy has in Chapter 10), and to work with people with intellectual disabilities and their families to maintain an effective lobby for good services in the community.

The second relevant influence is the integration of services for people with intellectual disabilities among other services. This is much more a feature of Sweden, Norway and Britain than of the United States. As several contributors to this book note there may be important disadvantages to such integration. These may include a weakening of commitment (especially when services for other client groups appear to be worse) or of expertise, as training and organizational procedures become more general and people with expertise in other areas take responsibility for intellectual disability services. It is too soon to tell whether the advantages of service integration outweigh these possible disadvantages. Study of this issue should therefore be a major item in the future research agenda, to understand the processes by which special needs are properly met without yielding the right of access to benefits available to everyone, i.e. how to achieve equality without invisibility. For the present discussion, though, it is enough to note that if 'dedifferentiation' leads to less commitment to, and competence in, providing good services this may threaten the policy of deinstitutionalization.

These different factors – costs, doubts about quality and integration of intellectual disability with other services – are likely to present continuing threats to deinstitutionalization. If it seems unlikely that any government in the countries studied would reverse the policy of 25 years it may still be worth while monitoring the interplay of pressures on policy.

The second question about the future is whether people with intellectual disabilities, their families and the staff who support them, will experience a better life in community services. There is evidence in all the countries studied of community services failing to break free from or reverting to institutional practices. Two different perspectives have been used to address this issue. Ericsson (Chapter 6) and Allard (Chapter 7) argue that the problem is located in the conceptualization of the service model and the role of the service user. They emphasize the definition of a new model (supported living) and a new role (citizen) as keys to the realization of good services in the community. Mansell (Chapter 4) and Felce (Chapter 8) focus on issues of training and management of the staff supporting people with intellectual disabilities as the key variables.

These are probably not mutually exclusive alternatives: ideology and philosophy is derived from, but also reinforces and extends, practice. There is a research and development agenda here, too, of continuing to try to understand the relationship between client needs and wishes, good care practices, service organization and management and wider social beliefs and views about intellectual disability, dependency and behaviour. In a sense, the study of institutions needs to continue even when the institutions have gone, to examine the origins of institutional practices and the conditions under which they become dominant. A significant part of this agenda should focus on staff and on family members, not only because these people have needs which ought to be met as well as those of service users but also because good services depend on a political and operational coalition between people with intellectual disabilities, their families and professionals.

Deinstitutionalization, then, is not just something that happened to people with intellectual disabilities and their families. It has also happened to decision-makers and staff in services and to researchers. They have had to shift their attention to new problems and issues in the community (such as many more problems of interorganizational work – at Castellani's 'seams of government'). But they have also to recognize that institutions were the expression of beliefs in society and that their demise may leave those beliefs and the practices they underpin still to be tackled in the community. This is surely the greatest challenge for all societies: how to build and sustain social solidarity and mutual commitment among people with different needs, talents and aspirations, so that everyone may flourish and prosper.

References

Abrahamsson, B. and Söder, M. (1979) Att förändra anstalter. *Psykisk Utvecklingshämning.* **81**(1), 1–6.

Agranoff, R.J. (1986) *Intergovernmental Management: Human Services Problem-Solving in Six Metropolitan Areas*, State University of New York Press, Albany, NY.

Aldrich, C.I. and Mendkoff, E. (1963) Relocation of the aged and disabled: A mortality study. *Journal of the American Geriatrics Society*, **11**, 185–194.

Allen, D. (1989) The effects of deinstitutionalisation on people with mental handicaps: A review. *Mental Handicap Research*, **2**, 18–37.

Allen, P., Pahl, J. and Quine, L. (1990) *Care Staff in Transition*, Her Majesty's Stationery Office, London.

Amado, A.N. and Heal, L. (eds) (1990) *Integration of Persons with Developmental Disabilities in the Community*, 2nd edn, Paul H. Brookes Publishing Co., Baltimore, MD.

American Association on Mental Retardation (1992) *Mental Retardation: Definition, Classification and Systems of Supports*, 9th edn, AAMR, Washington, DC.

Anderson, S.R. (1987) The management of staff behaviour in residential treatment facilities: A review of training techniques, in *Staff Training in Mental Handicap* (eds J. Hogg and P. Mittler), Croom Helm, Beckenham, pp.66–124.

Asplund, J. (1991) *Essä om Gemeinschaft och Gesellschaft*, Bokförlaget Korpen, Göteborg.

Audit Commission (1986) *Making a Reality of Community Care*, Her Majesty's Stationery Office, London.

Audit Commission (1987) *Community Care: Developing Services for People with a Mental Handicap. Occasional Paper No. 4*, Her Majesty's Stationery Office, London.

Ayer, S. and Alaszewski, A. (1984) *Community Care and the Mentally Handicapped: Services for Mothers and their Children*, Croom Helm, London.

Back, K.W. and Taylor, R.C. (1976) Self-help groups: Tool or symbol? *Journal of Applied Behavioral Science*, **12**, 295–309.

Balgopal, P. R., Ephross, P. H. and Vassil, T. V. (1986) Self-help groups and professional helpers. *Small Group Behavior*, **17**, 123–137.

Balla, D. (1976) Relationship of institution size to quality of care: A review of the literature. *American Journal of Mental Deficiency*, **81**, 117–124.

Bank-Mikkelsen, N.E. (1969) A Metropolitan Area in Denmark: Copenhagen, in *Changing Patterns in Residential Services for the Mentally Retarded* (eds R. Kugel and W. Wolfensberger), President's Committee on Mental Retardation, Washington, DC, pp.227–254.

Bardach, E. (1977) *The Implementation Game: What Happens After a Bill Becomes a Law*, The MIT Press, Cambridge, MA.

Beasley, F., Hewson, S. and Mansell, J. (1989) *MTS: Handbook for Observers*, Tizard Centre, University of Kent at Canterbury.

Bellah, R.H., Madsen, R., Sullivan, W.M. *et al.* (1985) *Habits of the Heart: Individualism and Commitment in American Life*, University of California Press, Berkeley, CA.

Bellah, R.H., Madsen, R., Sullivan, W.M. *et al.* (1991) *The Good Society*, Knopf, New York.

Bercovici, S.M. (1983) *Barriers to Normalization: The Restrictive Management of Mentally Retarded Persons*, University Park Press, Baltimore, MD.

Beswick, J. (1992) An Evaluation of the Effects on Quality of Life Outcome Measures for People with Learning Difficulties (Mental Handicap) of Changes in the Living Situation from Hospitals to Community Environments, University of Manchester, Manchester. Dissertation.

Beyer, S., Todd, S. and Felce, D. (1991) The implementation of the All Wales Mental Handicap Strategy, 1983–1988. *Mental Handicap Research*, **4**, 115–140.

Birenbaum, A. and Re, M. (1979) Resettling mentally retarded adults in the community: Almost 4 years later. *American Journal of Mental Deficiency*, **83**, 323–329.

Blunden, R. and Allen, D. (1987) *Facing the Challenge: An Ordinary Life for People with Learning Difficulties and Challenging Behaviours*, King's Fund, London.

Blunden, R. and Evans, G. (1988) Long-term maintenance of staff and resident behaviour in a hospital ward for adults with mental handicaps: Report of a six-year follow-up. *Mental Handicap Research*, **1**, 115–126.

Booth, T., Simons, S. and Booth, W. (1990) *Outward Bound*, Open University Press, Bristol.

Braddock, D. (1987) *Federal Policy Toward Mental Retardation and Developmental Disabilities*, Paul H. Brookes Publishing Co., Baltimore, MD.

Braddock, D., Hemp, R., Bachelder, L. and Fujiura, G. (1995) *The State of the States in Developmental Disabilities*, 4th edn, American Association on Mental Retardation, Washington, DC.

Braddock, D., Hemp, R., Fujiura, G. *et al.* (1990) *The State of the States in Developmental Disabilities*, Paul H. Brookes Publishing Co., Baltimore, MD.

Braddock, D. and Mitchell D. (1992) *Residential Services and Developmental Disabilities in the United States: A National Survey of Staff Compensation, Turnover and Related Issues*, American Association on Mental Retardation, Washington, DC.

Bradley, V.J. (1985) Implementation of court and consent decrees: Some current lessons, in *Living and Learning in the Least Restrictive Environment* (eds R.H. Bruininks and K.C. Lakin), Paul H. Brookes Publishing Co., Baltimore, MD, pp.81–96.

Bradley, V.J. and Knoll, J. (1991) *Shifting Paradigms in Services to People with Disabilities*, HSRI, Cambridge, MA.

Bradley, V.J. and Knoll, J.A. (1995) Shifting paradigms in services for people with developmental disabilities, in *The Community Revolution in Rehabilitation*

Services (eds O.C. Karan and S. Greenspan), Andover Press, Andover, MA.

Bradshaw, J., Glendinning, C. and Hatch, S. (1977) Voluntary organizations for handicapped children and their families: The meaning of membership. *Child: Care, Health and Development*, **3**, 247–260.

Bratt, A. and Johnston, R. (1988) Changes in lifestyle for young adults with profound handicaps following discharge from hospital care into a 'second generation' housing project. *Mental Handicap Research*, **1**, 49–74.

Brown, H. and Bailey, R. (1986) *Working with Families*. Bringing People Back Home: Series of video assisted training packages, Pavilion Publishing, Brighton.

Brown, H. and Bailey, R. (1987) *Participation in Everyday Activities*. Bringing People Back Home: Series of video assisted training packages, Bexhill; SETRHA, p.43.

Brown, H. and Smith, H. (1989) Whose ordinary life is it anyway? A feminist critique of community care policy. *Disability, Handicap and Society*, **4**, 105–120.

Brown, H. and Smith, H. (1993) Women caring for people: The mismatch between rhetoric and reality for women? *Policy and Politics*, **21**(3), 185–193.

Bruininks, R.H. (1990) There is more than a zip code to changes in services. *American Journal on Mental Retardation*, **95**, 13–15.

Bruininks, R.H., Kudla, M.J., Hauber, F.A. *et al.* (1981) Recent growth and status of community residential alternatives, in *Deinstitutionalization and Community Adjustment of Mentally Retarded People, AAMD Monograph No. 4.* (eds R.H. Bruininks *et al.*), American Association on Mental Deficiency, Washington, DC, pp.14–27.

Bruininks, R.H., Rotegard, L., Lakin, C. and Hill, B. (1987) Epidemiology of mental retardation and trends in residential services in the United States, in *Living Environments and Mental Retardation* (eds S. Landesman and P. Vietze), American Association on Mental Retardation, Washington, DC, pp.17–42.

Brusén, P. (1990) Avveckling utveckling. *PU-bladet*, **92**(4), 38–41.

Brusén, P. and Lerman, B. (1986) Institutionsavveckling – några erfarenheter. *Psykisk Utvecklingshämning*, **88**(2), 21–27.

Burg, M.M., Reid, D.H. and Lattimore, J. (1979) Use of a self-recording and supervision program to change institutional staff behavior. *Journal of Applied Behavior Analysis*, **12**, 363–375.

Burgess, P.M. (1975) Capacity building and the elements of public management. *Public Administration Review*, **35**(December), 705–716.

Burwell, B., Katz, R. and Allard, M. (1993) *Supported Living*, Assistant Secretary on Planning and Evaluation, US Department of Health and Human Services, Washington, DC, SysteMetrics, Lexington, MA.

Butler, E.W. and Bjaanes, A.T. (1977) A typology of community care facilities and differential normalization outcomes, in *Research to Practice in Mental Retardation*, volume 1, Care and Intervention (ed. P.Mittler), University Park Press, Baltimore, MD, pp.337–347.

Butterfield, E. (1987) Why and how to study the influence of living arrangements, in *Living Environments and Mental Retardation* (eds S. Landesman and P. Vietze), American Association on Mental Retardation, Washington, DC, pp.43–60.

California Department of Developmental Services (1978) The Client Development

Evaluation Report: Handbook, Sacramento: California Department of Developmental Services.

Cambridge, P., Hayes, L., Knapp, M. *et al.* (1994) *Care in the Community: Five Years On*, Ashgate Publishing Ltd, Aldershot.

Campaign for the Mentally Handicapped (1970) *Future services for the mentally handicapped: A manifesto*, Campaign for the Mentally Handicapped, London.

Campaign for the Mentally Handicapped (1972) *Even Better Services for the Mentally Handicapped*, Campaign for the Mentally Handicapped, London.

Cardiff and Vale of Glamorgan Community Health Councils (1977) *Future Services for Mentally Handicapped People in South Glamorgan (Report of a Shadow Health Care Planning Team chaired by J. Mansell)*, Cardiff and Vale of Glamorgan Community Health Councils, Cardiff.

Castellani, P.J. (1987) *The Political Economy of Developmental Disabilities*, Paul H. Brookes Publishing Co., Baltimore, MD.

Castellani, P.J. (1992) Closing institutions in New York State: Implementation and management lessons. *Journal of Policy Analysis and Management*, **11**(4), 593–611.

Castellani, P.J., Bird, W.A., Hanley, A.T. *et al.* (1990) *The Closure of Developmental Centers in New York State: Interim Report*, New York State Office of Mental Retardation and Developmental Disabilities, Albany, NY.

Cattermole, M., Jahoda, A. and Markova, I. (1988) Leaving home: The experience of people with a mental handicap. *Journal of Mental Deficiency Research*, **32**, 47–57.

Cochran, M. (1990) The transforming role. *Networking Bulletin*, **1**(3), 25.

Cochran, W.E., Sran, P.K. and Varano, G.A. (1977) The relocation syndrome in the mentally retarded. *Mental Retardation*, **15**, 10–12.

Coffman, T.L. (1981) Relocation and survival of institutionalized aged: A re-examination of the evidence. *The Gerontologist*, **21**, 483–500.

Cohen, S. (1985) *Visions of Social Control*, Polity Press, Oxford.

Cohen, H., Conroy, J.W., Frazer, D.W. *et al.* (1977) Behavioral effects of interinstitutional relocation of mentally retarded residents. *American Journal of Mental Deficiency*, **82**, 12–18.

Coles, R. (1993) *The Call for Service*, Houghton Mifflin, Boston, MA.

Committee on Handicap Services (1981) SOU 1981:26: Omsorger om vissa handikappade. Betänkande från Omsorgskommittén. Stockholm: Socialdepartementet.

Conneally, S., Boyle, G. and Smyth, F. (1992) An evaluation of the use of small group homes for adults with a severe and profound mental handicap. *Mental Handicap Research*, **5**, 146–168.

Connecticut Department of Mental Retardation (1987) *Mission Statement*, Department of Mental Retardation, Hartford, CN.

Conroy, J. (1992) *1992 Survey of the Families of the Former Residents of Johnstone Training and Research Center: Their Opinions About the Well-Being of Their Relatives. The New Jersey Strategic Planning Project, Report Number 4*, PA: Conroy and Feinstein Associates, Wynnewood.

Conroy, J. (1994) *The Small ICF/MR Program: Dimensions of Quality and Cost*, PA: Conroy and Feinstein Associates, Wynnewood.

Conroy, J. and Bradley, V.J. (1985) The Pennhurst Longitudinal Study: A Report of Five Years of Research and Analysis, Temple University Developmental

Disabilities Center, Philadelphia, PA.

Conroy, J. and Feinstein, C. (1990a) A new way of thinking about quality, in *Quality Assurance for Individuals with Developmental Disabilities: It's Everybody's Business* (eds V.J. Bradley and H.A. Bersani), Paul H. Brookes Publishing Co., Baltimore, MD, pp.263–278.

Conroy, J. and Feinstein, C. (1990b) Measuring quality of life: Where have we been? Where are we going?, in *Quality of Life: Perspectives and Issues*, Monograph No. 12 (eds R. Schalock and M. Begab), American Association on Mental Retardation, Washington, DC, pp.227–234.

Conroy, J. and Seiders, J. (1994) *1993 Report on the Well-Being of the Former Residents of Johnstone Training and Research Centre, The New Jersey Strategic Planning Project, Report Number 5*, PA: Conroy and Feinstein Associates, Wynnewood.

Craig, E.M. and McCarver, R.B. (1984) Community placement and adjustment for deinstitutionalised clients: Issues and findings, in *International Review of Research in Mental Retardation*, volume 12 (eds N. Ellis and N. Bray), Academic Press Inc, Orlando, pp.95–122.

Croser, M.D. (1995) Perspectives: Word from Washington. *Mental Retardation*, 33(1), 49–53.

Cullen, C., Burton, M., Watts, S. and Thomas, M. (1983) A preliminary report of interactions in a mental handicap institution. *Behaviour Research and Therapy*, 21, 579–583.

Dailey, W.F., Allen, G.J., Chinsky, J.M. and Veit, S.W. (1974) Attendant behavior and attitudes toward institutionalized retarded children. *American Journal of Mental Deficiency*, 78, 586–591.

Dam, A. (1985) Fra omklaring til aktiv medleven. *Psykisk Utvecklingshämning*, 87(3), 15–18.

Dam, A., Lunde, R., Sletved, H. and Haubro, H. (1982) *Hvad Gör Vi Med De Store Institutioner?* Imprint, Naestved.

Darling, R.B. (1988) Parental entrepreneurship: A consumerist response to professional dominance. *Journal of Social Issues*, 44, 141–158.

Davies, L. (1988) Community care: The costs and quality. *Health Services Management Research*, 1, 145–155.

Davies, B. and Challis, D. (1986) *Matching Resources to Needs in Community Care*, Gower Publishing Company Ltd, Aldershot.

de Kock, U., Saxby, H., Thomas, M. and Felce, D. (1988) Community and family contact: An evaluation of small community homes for adults with severe and profound mental handicaps. *Mental Handicap Research*, 1, 127–140.

de Kock, U., Saxby, H., Felce, D. *et al.* (1988) Community and family contact: An evaluation of small community homes for severely and profoundly mentally handicapped adults, *Mental Handicap*, 1, 127–140.

Department of Health (1989a) *Needs and Responses*, Department of Health, London.

Department of Health (1989b) *Caring for People: Community Care in the Next Decade and Beyond*, Her Majesty's Stationery Office, London.

Department of Health (1992) *Social Care for Adults with Learning Disabilities (Mental Handicap)* Local Authority Circular LAC(92)15, Department of Health, London.

Department of Health (1993) *Services for People with Learning Disabilities and*

Challenging Behaviour or Mental Health Needs: Report of a Project Group (Chairman: Prof. J.L. Mansell), Her Majesty's Stationery Office: London.

Department of Health and Social Security (1971) *Better Services for the Mentally Handicapped* (Cmnd 4683), Her Majesty's Stationery Office, London.

Department of Health and Social Security (1984) *Helping Mentally Handicapped People with Special Problems,* Her Majesty's Stationery Office, London.

Derby, K.M., Wacker, D.P., Sasso, G. *et al.* (1992) Brief functional assessment techniques to evaluate aberrant behavior in an outpatient setting: A summary of 79 cases. *Journal of Applied Behavior Analysis,* **25,** 713–721.

Design for Special Needs (1977) *Two Ordinary Terraced Houses in Skelmersdale Adapted to House Six Mentally Handicapped Children and Two Houseparents, January–April,* pp.10–13.

Devlin, S. (1989) *Reliability Assessment of the Instruments used to Monitor the Pennhurst Plaintiff Class Members,* Temple University Developmental Disabilities Center/University Affiliated Program, Philadelphia.

Di Terlizzi, M. (1994) Life history: The impact of a changing service provision on an individual with learning disabilities. *Disability and Society,* **9**(4), 501–517.

Dockrell, J., Gaskell, G., Rehman. H. and Normand, C. (1993) Service provision for people with mild learning difficulty and challenging behaviours: The MIETS evaluation, in *Research To Practice? Implications of Research on the Challenging Behaviour of People with Learning Disabilities* (ed. C. Kiernan), British Institute of Learning Disabilities, Clevedon, pp.245–270.

Drake, R.F. (1992) Consumer participation: The voluntary sector and the concept of power. *Disability, Handicap and Society,* **7,** 267–278.

Dufresne, D. (1992) Current issues in residential services, in *Supported Living Monograph,* volume 2, National Association of Private Residential Resources, Arlington, VA, pp.111–119.

Duker, P.C., Boonekamp, J., Brummelhuis, Y.T. *et al.* (1989) Analysis of ward staff initiatives towards mentally retarded residents: Clues for intervention. *Journal of Mental Deficiency Research,* **33,** 55–67.

Duker, P.C., Seys, D., Leeuwe, J.V. and Prins, L.W. (1991) Occupational conditions of ward staff and quality of residential care for individuals with mental retardation. *American Journal on Mental Retardation,* **95,** 388–396.

Durkheim, E. (1915) *The Elementary Forms of Religious Life,* Allen and Unwin, London.

Ebenstein, W. and Gooler, L. (1993) *Cultural Diversity and Developmental Disabilities Workforce Issues,* The City University of New York Consortium for the Study of Disabilities, New York, NY.

Edgerton, R. (1967) *The Cloak of Competence,* University of California Press, Berkeley, CA.

Edgerton, R., Bollinger, M. and Herr, B. (1984) The cloak of competence: After two decades. *American Journal of Mental Deficiency,* **88,** 345–351.

Elmore, R.F. (1986) Graduate education in public management: Working the seams of government. *Journal of Policy Analysis and Management,* **6**(1), 69–83.

Emerson, E. (1985) Evaluating the impact of deinstitutionalization on the lives of mentally retarded people. *American Journal of Mental Deficiency,* **90,** 277–288.

Emerson, E. (1990) Designing individualised community based placements as alternatives to institutions for people with a severe mental handicap and severe problem behaviour, in *Key Issues in Mental Retardation Research* (ed. W. Fraser), Routledge, London, pp.395–404.

Emerson, E. (1992) What is normalisation? in *Normalisation: A Reader for the 1990s* (eds H. Smith and H. Brown), Routledge, London.

Emerson, E., Beasley, F., Offord, G. and Mansell, J. (1992) Specialised housing for people with seriously challenging behaviours. *Journal of Mental Deficiency Research*, **36**, 291–307.

Emerson, E., Cambridge, P., Forrest, J. and Mansell, J. (1993) Community support teams for people with learning disabilities and challenging behaviours, in *Research into Practice? Implications of Research on the Challenging Behaviour of People with Learning Disabilities* (ed. C. Kiernan), British Institute of Learning Disabilities, Kidderminster, pp.229–243.

Emerson, E., Cooper, J., Hatton, C. et al. (1993) *An Evaluation of the Quality and Costs of Residential Further Education Services Provided by SENSE-Midlands*, Hester Adrian Research Centre, Manchester.

Emerson, E. and Hatton, C. (1994) *Moving Out: Re-location from Hospital to Community*, Her Majesty's Stationery Office, London.

Emerson, E. and McGill, P. (1989) Normalisation and applied behaviour analysis: Values and technology in services for people with learning difficulties. *Behavioural Psychotherapy*, **17**, 101–117.

Emerson, E. and McGill, P. (1993) Developing services for people with severe learning disabilities and seriously challenging behaviours: South East Thames Regional Health Authority, 1985–1991, in *People with Learning Disability and Severe Challenging Behaviour* (eds I. Fleming and B. Stenfert Kroese), Manchester University Press, Manchester, pp.83–113.

Engberg, M. (1982) Afdelningernes selvstaendiggörelse. *Psykisk Utvecklings-hämning*, **84**(4), 10–14.

Ericsson, K. (1981) Normativ modell, beskrivning och utvärdering av dagcenter-verksamhet, in *Evaluering av Öppna Omsorgsformer* (eds L. Kebbon et al.), Liber Förlag, Stockholm, pp.152–204.

Ericsson, K. (1985a) The origin and consequences of the normalization principle. Paper presented at the *International Association for the Scientific Study of Mental Deficiency Conference*, New Delhi.

Ericsson, K. (1985b) From institutional to community life: Towards a normal way of life for the intellectually handicapped person, in *Growing in Wisdom – The Mentally Retarded Person in Asia, Proceedings of 7th Asian Conference on Mental Retardation* (ed. B. O'Connell), Asian Federation for the Mentally Retarded, Taipei, pp.179–183.

Ericsson, K.(1986a) Omsorger för förståndshandikappades samhällsdeltagande. *Socialmedicinsk Tidskrift*, nr1–2, pp.11–16.

Ericsson, K. (1986b) Der Normalisieringungsgedanke: Entstehung und erfarungen in Skandinavischen ländern, in Normalisierung: *Eine chance fur Menschen mit Geistiger Behinderung* (ed. S. Bothe), Marburg/Lahn: Lebenshilfe, pp.33–44.

Ericsson, K. (1987a) Normalization: History and experiences in Scandinavian countries. *Superintendent's Digest*, **6**(4), 124–130.

Ericsson, K. (1987b) *Anhöriga Flyttar*, Centre for Handicap Research, Uppsala University.

Ericsson, K. et al. (1987) Förståndshandikappade flyttar: Personlig utveckling och vårdhemsavveckling. *Social Forskning*.

Ericsson, K. (1989) Omsorgernas förändring på de utvecklingsstördas villkor. Ur *Sävstaholmssymposium: Vad innebär dagens forsknings- och utvecklingsarbete för den utvecklingsstörde år 1998?* Stockholm: Sävstaholmsföreningen.

Ericsson, K. (1990) Dagliga omsorger för samhällsdeltagande. Ur Ericsson and Nilsson: *Dagliga verksamheter i kommunal regi för vuxna personer med begåvningshandikapp.* Rapport. Uppsala: Projekt Mental Retardation, Uppsala Universitet, pp.116–157.

Ericsson, K. (1991) *Den goda gruppbostaden*, Rapport. Uppsala: Skinfaxe Institute.

Ericsson, K. (1993) *Esfer att ha flyttat från Carlslund.* En uppföljning efter ett vårdhems avveckling, Centre for Handicap Research, Uppsala University.

Ericsson, K. (1994) *Ny vardag och nya livsvilkor. Efter avveckling av vårdhem för utvecklingsstörda i Skaraborg,* Centre for Handicap Research, Uppsala University.

Ericsson, K., Enarsson, S., Mehlberg, L. and Schultz, T. (1983) Avvecklingsplan för ett vårdhem. *Psykisk Utvecklingshämning,* 85(2), 20–27.

Ericsson, K. and Ericsson, P. (1980) *Två synsätt på boende för personer med förståndshandikapp.* FUB:s föredragsserie nr 4. Stockholm: Riksförbundet FUB.

Ericsson, P. and Ericsson, K. (1988) Community services: Housing and a home, in *Intellectual Disability: Perspectives and Challenges* (ed. F. Chen), Committee for the Promotion of Services for the Intellectually Disabled, Singapore, pp.396–402.

Ericsson, K. and Ericsson, P. (1989) Two perspectives on the life of the person with intellectual handicap, in *Quality of Life for the Mentally Retarded, Proceedings from 9th Asian Conference on Mental Retardation,* The Foundation for the Welfare of the Mentally Retarded of Thailand, Bangkok, pp.607–616.

Ericsson, K., Thorsell, M. and Widman, E. (1980) Behov av alternativa omsorger efter utflyttning från Carlslund och Klockbacka. Del 1. Resurser för boende, dagliga verksamheter och fritid för Carlslunds och Klockbackas omsorgstagare. Ur *Enarsson, S. et al. 1981: Plan för Carlslunds och Klockbackas avveckling.* Stockholm: Omsorgsnämnden.

Esping-Andersen, G. (1990) *The Three Worlds of Welfare Capitalism,* Polity Press, Oxford.

Etzioni, A. (1993) *The Spirit of Community: Rights, Responsibilities and the Communitarian Agenda,* Crown, New York.

Farmer, R., Rohde, J. and Sacks, B. (1991) *Dimensions of Mental Handicap: A Study of People with Mental Handicaps in the North West Thames Region,* Charing Cross and Westminster Medical School, London.

Fasting, A.F. (1987) Institusjonsavvikling i Norge. *Psykisk Utvecklingshämning,* 89(4), 33–37.

Felce, D. (1988) Behavioral and social climate in community group residences, in *Community Residences for Persons with Developmental Disabilities: Here to Stay* (eds M.P. Janicki, M.W. Krauss and M.M. Seltzer), Paul H. Brookes Publishing Co., Baltimore, MD, pp.133–147.

Felce, D. (1989) *The Andover Project: Staffed Housing for Adults with Severe or Profound Mental Handicaps,* British Institute on Mental Handicap, Kidderminster.

Felce, D. (1991) Using behavioural principles in the development of effective housing services for adults with severe or profound handicap, in *The Challenge of Severe Mental Handicap: A Behaviour Analytic Approach* (ed. B.

Remington), Wiley, Chichester, pp.285–316.

Felce, D. (1993) Is community care expensive? The costs and benefits of residential models for people with severe mental handicaps. *Mental Handicap*, **21**, 2–6.

Felce, D., de Kock, U. and Repp, A.C. (1986) An eco-behavioral comparison of small home and institutional settings for severely and profoundly mentally handicapped adults. *Applied Research in Mental Retardation*, **7**, 393–408.

Felce, D., de Kock, U., Thomas, M. and Saxby, H. (1986) Change in adaptive behaviour of severely and profoundly mentally handicapped adults in different residential settings, *British Journal of Psychology*, **77**, 489–501.

Felce, D., Kushlick, A. and Smith, J. (1980) An overview of the research on alternative residential facilities for the severely mentally handicapped in Wessex. *Advances in Behaviour Research and Therapy*, **3**, 1–4.

Felce, D., Kushlick, A. and Mansell, J. (1980a) Evaluation of alternative residential facilities for the severely mentally handicapped in Wessex: Client engagement. *Advances in Behaviour Research and Therapy*, **3**, 13–18.

Felce, D., Kushlick, A. and Mansell, J. (1980b) Evaluation of alternative residential facilities for the severely mentally handicapped in Wessex: Staff recruitment and continuity. *Advances in Behaviour Research and Therapy*, **3**, 31–35.

Felce, D., Mansell, J. and Kushlick, A. (1980a) Evaluation of alternative residential facilities for the severely mentally handicapped in Wessex: Revenue costs. *Advances in Behaviour Research and Therapy*, **3**, 43–47.

Felce, D., Mansell, J. and Kushlick, A. (1980b) Evaluation of alternative residential facilities for the severely mentally handicapped in Wessex: Staff performance. *Advances in Behaviour Research and Therapy*, **3**, 25–30.

Felce, D. and Repp, A.C. (1992) Behavioral and social climate of community residences. *Research in Developmental Disabilities*, **13**, 27–42.

Felce, D., Repp, A.C., Thomas, M. *et al.* (1991) The relationship of staff:client ratios, interactions and residential placement. *Research in Developmental Disabilities*, **12**, 315–331.

Felce, D., Saxby, H., de Kock, U. *et al.* (1987) To what behaviors do attending adults respond? A replication. *American Journal of Mental Deficiency*, **91**, 496–504.

Felce, D., Thomas, M., de Kock, U. *et al.* (1985) An ecological comparison of small community-based houses and traditional institutions: Physical setting and the use of opportunities. *Behaviour Research and Therapy*, **23**, 337–348.

Felce, D. and Toogood, S. (1988) *Close to Home*, British Institute of Mental Handicap, Kidderminster.

Ferguson, P.M., Hibbard, M., Leinen, J. and Schaff, S. (1990) Supported community life: Disability policy and the renewal of mediating structure. *Journal of Disability Policy Studies*. **1**(1), 9–35.

Fleming, I. and Stenfert Kroese, B. (1990) Evaluation of a community care project for people with learning difficulties. *Journal of Mental Deficiency Research*, **34**, 451–464.

Foucault, M. (1961) *Folie et déraison*. Librairie Plon, Paris.

Foucault, M. (1967) *Madness and Civilization*, Tavistock Publications Ltd, London.

Freeman, M. (1993) Evaluation of a Training Programme for Carers Working in Community Homes for those with Learning Difficulties, University of Sussex, Brighton. Dissertation.

Frohboese, R. and Sales, B.D. (1980) Parental opposition to deinstitutionalisation: A challenge in need of attention and resolution. *Law and Human Behavior*, **4**, 1–87.

Gardner, J.F. (1992) Quality, organizational design and standards. *Mental Retardation*. **30**(3), 173–177.

Gargan, J.J. (1981) Consideration of local government capacity. *Public Administration Review*, (November/December), 649–658.

Gartner, A. and Riessman, F. (1977) *Self-help in the Human Services*, Jossey-Bass, San Francisco.

Gettings, R.M. (1992a) Responding to a changing policymaking and programmatic environment. Keynote address to the *North Carolina Council of Community Mental Health, Developmental Disabilities and Substance Abuse*, May.

Gettings, R. (July 22, 1992b) CSLA evaluation project, *Memorandum to Ruth Katz, U.S.DHHS. ASPE.*, U.S. DHHS, ASPE, Washington, DC.

Goffman, E. (1961) *Asylums*. Doubleday & Co., New York.

Goggin, M.L., Bowman, A. O'M., Lester, J.P. and O'Toole, L.J. Jr (1990) *Implementation Theory and Practice: Toward a Third Generation*, Scott, Foresman Co., Glenview, IL.

Goldsmith, M. and Newton, K. (1988) Centralization and decentralization: Changing patterns of intergovernmental relations in advanced western societies. *European Journal of Political Research*, **16**(4), 359–363.

Gourash, N. (1978) Help-seeking: A review of the literature. *American Journal of Psychology*, **6**, 413–423.

Grant, G.W.B. and Moores, B. (1977) Resident characteristics and staff behavior in two hospitals for mentally retarded adults. *American Journal of Mental Deficiency*, **82**, 259–265.

Greig, R. (1993) The replacement of hospital services with community services based on individual need. Paper presented at the *Hester Adrian Research Centre Conference on Hospital Closure*, Manchester, November 1993.

Griffiths, R. (1988) *Community Care: Agenda for Action*, Her Majesty's Stationery Office, London.

Gross. E. and Etzioni, A. (1985) *Organizations in Society*, Prentice-Hall, Englewood Cliffs, NJ.

Grunewald, K. (1987) Avveckling genom utveckling. *Psykisk Utvecklingshämning*, **89**(2), 1–16.

Grunewald, K. (1992) Den lilla gruppens princip. *Intra B/92*, 9–11.

Gustavsson, A. and Söder, M. (1990) *Social forskning om människor med psykisk utvecklingsstörning*, Vårdhøgskölan i Stockholm, FoU-rapport 1990:1.

Gustavsson, A. (1990) *Difficulties and opportunities for people with disabilities living in integrated society: Scandinavian experiences*. Stockholm College of Health and Caring Sciences, Stockholm.

Guy's Health District (1981) *Development Group for Services for Mentally Handicapped People: Report to the District Management Team*, Guy's Health District, London.

Halpern, A.S., Close, D.W. and Nelson, D.J. (1986) *On Our Own*, Paul H. Brookes Publishing Co., Baltimore, MD.

Haney, J.I. (1988) Toward successful community residential placements for individuals with mental retardation, in *Integration of Developmentally Disabled Individuals into the Community*, 2nd edn (eds L.W. Heal, J.I. Haney, A.R.N.

Amado), Paul H. Brookes Publishing Co., Baltimore, MD, pp.37–58.

Hansen, J. (1978) Kan store institutioner 'aftotaliseres'? *Psykisk Utvecklingshämning*, **80**(2), 10–13.

Harris, C. (1982) An Interrater Reliability Study of the Client Development Evaluation Report. Final Report to the California Department of Developmental Services.

Harris, J.M., Veit, S.W., Allen G.J. and Chinsky, J.M. (1974) Aide:resident ratio and ward population density as mediators of social interaction. *American Journal of Mental Deficiency*, **79**, 320–326.

Harsheim, J. and Sandvin, J. (1991) *Organisering i kommunene – vilje til endring*, NIBR/Nordlandsforskning.

Hautamäki, J. (1987) Avveckling av institutioner som ett socialpolitiskt program. *Psykisk Utvecklingshämning*, **89**(4), 11–16.

Heal, L.W. (1987) Institutions cost more than community services. *American Journal of Mental Deficiency*, **92**(2), 136–138.

Heller, T. (1982) Social disruption and residential relocation of mentally retarded children. *American Journal of Mental Deficiency*, **87**, 48–55.

Heller, T. (1984) Issues in adjustment of mentally retarded individuals to residential relocation. *International Review of Research in Mental Retardation*, **12**, 123–147.

Heller, T. (1988) Transitions: Coming in and going out of community residences, in *Community Residences for Persons with Developmental Disabilities* (eds M.P. Janicki, M.W. Krauss and M.M. Seltzer), Paul H. Brookes Publishing Co., Baltimore, MD, pp.149–158.

Heller, T., Bond, M. and Braddock, D. (1988) Family reactions to institutional closure. *American Journal on Mental Retardation*, **92**, 336–343.

Hemming, H., Castell, J., Cook, M. and Pill, R. (1979) *A Real Home Life: A Study of Purpose-built Residential Units for Mentally Handicapped Adults*, Department of Social Administration, University College of Swansea, Swansea.

Hemming, H., Lavender, T. and Pill, R. (1981) Quality of life of mentally retarded adults transferred from large institutions to new small units. *American Journal of Mental Deficiency*, **86**, 157–169.

Hemming, M. (1982) Mentally handicapped adults returned to large institutions after transfers to new small units. *British Journal of Mental Subnormality*, **5**, 13–28.

Heron, A. and Phillips, J. (1977) *The Sheffield Development Project on Services for the Mentally Handicapped: Implementation of the Feasibility Study Recommendations*, University of Sheffield, Sheffield.

Herr, S. (1992) Beyond benevolence: Legal protection for persons with special needs, in *Mental Retardation in the Year 2000* (ed. L. Rowitz), Springer-Verlag, New York, pp.279–298.

Hewson, S. and Walker, J. (1992) The use of evaluation in the development of a staffed residential service for adults with mental handicap. *Mental Handicap Research*, **5**, 188–203.

Holburn, C.S. (1992) Symposium overview: Are we making the same mistake twice? *Mental Retardation*, **30**(3), 129–132.

Horner, R.D. (1980) The effects of an environmental 'enrichment' program on the behavior of institutionalized profoundly retarded children. *Journal of Applied*

Behavior Analysis, **13**, 473–491.

House of Commons Social Services Committee (1985) *Community Care: With Special Reference to Adult Mentally Ill and Mentally Handicapped People*, Her Majesty's Stationery Office, London.

Hunter, D.J. and Wistow, G. (1987) *Community Care in Britain: Variations on a Theme*, King's Fund, London.

Intagliata, J. and Willer, B. (1982) Reinstitutionalisation of mentally retarded persons successfully placed into family-care and group homes. *American Journal of Mental Deficiency*, **87**(1), 34–39.

Janicki, M.P. (1981) Personal growth and community residence environments: A review, in *Living Environments for Developmentally Retarded Persons* (eds H.C. Haywood and J.R. Newbrough), University Park Press, Baltimore, MD.

Jasnau, K.F. (1967) Individualized vs. mass transfer on non-psychotic geriatric patients from mental hospitals to nursing homes with special reference to death rate. *Journal of the American Geriatrics Society*, **15**, 280–284.

Jensen, K. (1992) *Hjemlig omsorg i offentlig regi*, Universitetsforlaget, Oslo.

Johnson, T. (1985) *Belonging to the Community*, Options in Community Living and the Wisconsin Developmental Disabilities Planning Council, Madison, WI.

Kaipio, K. (1983) Ansvarspedagogik på anstalt. *Psykisk Utvecklingshämning*, **85**(3), 34–39.

Kalifon, S.Z. (1991) Self-help groups providing services: Conflict and change. *Nonprofit and Voluntary Sector Quarterly*, **20**, 191–205.

Karan, O.C. and Granfield, J.M. (1990) *Engaging people in life: A report on one supported living program in Connecticut*, Pappankiou Center on Special Education and Rehabilitation, University Affiliated Program, East Hartford, CN.

Karan, O.C., Granfield, J.M. and Furey, E.M. (1992) Supported living: Rethinking the rules of residential services. *Amercian Association on Mental Retardation News and Notes*, **5**(1), 5.

Katz, A.H. (1961) *Parents of the Handicapped*, Charles C. Thomas, Springfield, IL.

Katz, A.H. (1981) Self-help and mutual aid: An emerging social movement? *Annual Review of Sociology*, **7**, 129–155.

Katz, A.H. and Bender, E.I. (eds) (1976) *The Strength in Us: Self-help Groups in the Modern World*, New Viewpoints, New York.

Kebbon, L. (1979) Perspectives on Mental Retardation, in *Three Papers – International Association for the Scientific Study of Mental Deficiency Congress, Jerusalem*, Uppsala: Projekt Mental Retardation, Uppsala Universitet, pp.1–13.

Kendrick, M. (1989) Some reflections on community living reform and personal conduct. *Interaction*, **3**, 19–27.

Killilea, M. (1976) Mutual help organizations: Interpretations in the literature, in *Support Systems and Mutual Help: Multidisciplinary Explorations* (eds G. Caplan and M. Killilea), Grune & Stratton Inc, New York, pp.37–93.

King, R., Raynes, N. and Tizard, J. (1971) *Patterns of Residential Care: Sociological Studies in Institutions for Handicapped Children*, Routledge & Kegan Paul, London.

King's Fund (1980) *An Ordinary Life: Comprehensive Locally-Based Residential Services for Mentally Handicapped People*, King's Fund Centre, London.

King's Fund (1984) *An Ordinary Working Life: Vocational Services for People with Mental Handicap*, King's Fund Centre, London.

King's Fund (1989) *An Ordinary Life and Treatment under Security for People with Mental Health*, King's Fund Centre, London.

Kingdon, J.W. (1987) *Agendas, Alternatives and Public Policies*, Little, Brown & Co., Boston, MA.

Klein, J. (1991) Supported living: The answer (no), a value (yes). *The New Hampshire Challenge*, 3(4), 1–2.

Klein, J. (1992) Get me the hell out of here: Supporting people with disabilities to live in their own homes, in *Natural Supports in School Work and Community* (ed. J. Nisbet), Paul H. Brookes Publishing Co., Baltimore, MD, pp.277–339.

Kleinberg, J. and Galligan, B. (1983) Effects of deinstitutionalization on adaptive behaviour of mentally retarded adults. *American Journal of Mental Deficiency*, 88, 21–27.

Knapp, M., Cambridge, P., Thomason, C. et al. (1992) *Care in the Community. Challenge and Demonstration*, Ashgate, Aldershot.

Knoll, J. (1992) What does it mean to provide support? Paper presented at the *Annual Public Policy Forum*, American Association on Mental Retardation, Washington, DC, 8 December.

Knoll, J.A. and Racino, J.A. (1994) Field in search of a home, in *Creating Individual Supports for People with Developmental Disabilities: A Mandate for Change at Many Levels* (eds V.J. Bradley, J.W. Ashbaugh and B.C. Blaney), Paul H. Brookes Publishing Co., Baltimore, MD.

Kommittén för partiellt arbetsföra, (1949) Partiellt arbetsföras problem. En översikt över kommitténs för partiellt arbetsföra förslag. Stockholm: Arbetsmarknadsstyrelsen.

Korman, N. and Glennerster, H. (1985) *Closing a Hospital: The Darenth Park Project*, Bedford Square Press, London.

Korman, N. and Glennerster, H. (1990) *Hospital Closure*, Open University Press, Milton Keynes.

Kugel, R. and Wolfensberger, W. (1969) Why innovate action?, in *Changing Patterns in Residential Services for the Mentally Retarded* (eds R. Kugel and W. Wolfensberger), President's Committee on Mental Retardation, Washington, DC, pp.1–14.

Kuhnle, S. (1990) The Scandinavian Welfare Model in the era of European integration: Some thoughts on internal and external pressure for change. Paper presented at *ECPR Joint Sessions of Workshops*, Ruhr-Universität Bochum, April.

Kurtz, L.F. (1990) The self-help movement: Review of the past decade of research. *Social Work with Groups*, 13, 101–115.

Kylén, G. (1972) Målsättningsanalys av boende. *Psykisk Utvecklingshämning*, 74(2), 1–6.

Lakin, K.C., Bruininks, R.H. and Sigford, B.H. (1981) Introduction, in *Deinstitutionalization and Community Adjustment of Mentally Retarded People*, AAMD Monograph No. 4 (eds R.H. Bruininks et al.) American Association on Mental Deficiency, Washington, DC, pp.vii–xvi.

Lakin, K.C., Hill, B.K. and Bruininks, R.H. (1988) Trends and issues in the growth of community residential services, in *Community Residences for People with Developmental Disabilities: Here to Stay* (eds M. Janicki, M. Krauss and M. Seltzer), Paul H. Brookes Publishing Co., Baltimore, MD, pp.25–42.

Lakin, K.C., Jaskulski, T.M., Hill, B.K. et al. (1989) *Medicaid Services for Persons with*

Mental Retardation and Related Conditions, University of Minnesota, Institute on Community Integration, Minneapolis.

Landesman, S. (1988) Preventing 'institutionalisation' in the community, in *Community Residences for Persons with Developmental Disabilities: Here to Stay* (eds M.P. Janicki, M.W. Krauss and M.M. Seltzers), Paul H. Brookes Publishing Co., Baltimore, MD, pp.105–116.

Landesman, S. and Butterfield, E. (1987) Normalization and deinstitutionalization of mentally retarded individuals. *American Psychologist*, **42**, 809–816.

Landesman-Dwyer, S. (1981) Living in the community. *American Journal of Mental Deficiency*, **86**, 223–234.

Landesman-Dwyer, S., Sackett G. and Kleinman, J. (1980) Relationship of size to resident and staff behavior in small community residences. *American Journal of Mental Deficiency*, **85**, 6–17.

Langer, M., Agosta, J. and Choisser, L. (1988) *Proposed Model for a State-Sponsored Direct Care Staff Training System in Iowa: Final Report*, Human Services Research Institute, Cambridge, MA.

Larson, S.A., Hewitt, A. and Lakin, C.K. (1994) Residential services personnel: Recruitment, training and retention, in *Challenges for a Service System in Transition: Ensuring Quality Community Experiences for Persons with Developmental Disabilities* (eds M. Hayden and B. Abery), Paul H. Brookes Publishing Co., Baltimore, MD.

Larson, S.A. and Lakin, K.C. (1989) Deinstitutionalization of persons with mental retardation: Behavioral outcomes. *Journal of the Association for Persons with Severe Disabilities*, **14**, 324–332.

Larson, S.A. and Lakin, K.C. (1991) Parent attitudes about residential placement before and after deinstitutionalization: a research synthesis. *Journal of the Association for Persons with Severe Handicaps*, **16**, 25–38.

Laski, F. (1980) Right to services in the community: Implications of the Pennhurst case, in *Normalization, Social Integration and Community Services* (eds R.J. Flynn and K.E. Nitsch), University Park Press, Baltimore, pp.167–185.

Latib, A., Conroy, J. and Hess, C. (1984) Family attitudes toward deinstitutionalization, in *International Review of Research in Mental Retardation*, volume 12 (eds N. Ellis and N. Bray), Academic Press, New York, pp.67–93.

Lazarus, R.S. and Folkman, S. (1984) *Stress, Appraisal and Coping*, Springer, New York.

Lemanowicz, J., Levine, R., Feinstein, C. and Conroy, J. (1990) Evaluation of the well being of non class members living in the community in 1990; the results of Temple monitoring in Philadelphia. Project Report **19**, 2 to the Philadelphia Office of Mental Health and Mental Retardation, Philadelphia; Temple University Developmental Disabilities Center/UAP.

Lentz, R.J. and Paul, G.L. (1971) 'Routine' vs. 'therapeutic' transfer of chronic mental patients. *Archives of General Psychiatry*, **25**, 187–191.

Levin, M.A. (1993) The day after an AIDS vaccine is discovered: Management matters. *Journal of Policy Analysis and Managment*, **12**(3), 438–455.

Levy, L. (1976) Self-help groups: Types and psychological processes. *Journal of Applied Behavioral Science*, **12**, 310–322.

Lieberson, S. (1985) *Making it Count*, University of California Press, Berkeley, CA.

Lindman, C. (1982) Vårdhemmens inre arbete. *Psykisk Utvecklingshämning*, **84**(4), 26–37.

Løchen, Y. (1990) Den sosiale forvitringen, in *Formål og Fellesskap* (ed. Løchen), Oslo.

Lowe, K. and de Paiva, S.D. (1990) *The Evaluation of NIMROD, A Community Based Service for People with Mental Handicap: Changes in Clients' Skill Levels and Usage*, Mental Handicap in Wales – Applied Research Unit, Cardiff.

Lowe, K. and de Paiva, S.D. (1991) *NIMROD: An Overview. A Summary Report of a 5 Year Research Study of Community Based Service Provision for People with Learning Difficulties*, Her Majesty's Stationery Office, London.

Lund, R.B. (1992) *Planlagt og iverksatt?* NF-rapport nr38/92–60.

Lynn, L.E. Jr (1981) *Managing the Public's Business: The Job of the Government Executive*, Basic Books, New York.

MacNamara, R.D. (1994) The Mansfield Training School is closed: The swamp has been finally drained. *Mental Retardation*, **32**(3), 239–242.

Malin, N.A. (1982) Group homes for mentally handicapped adults: residents' views on contact and support. *British Journal of Mental Subnormality*, **28**, 29–34.

Malin, N.A. (1987) (ed.) *Reassessing Community Care*, Croom Helm, London.

Mansell, J. (1976) Students show the way, *New Psychiatry*. **3**, 12–13.

Mansell, J. (1977) CUSS – A student project at University College Cardiff, in *Involvement of the Client, the Family and the Community: Report of the Tenth Spring Conference on Mental Retardation*, National Society for Mentally Handicapped Children, Exeter, pp.39–51.

Mansell, J. (1980) Susan: The successful resolution of a severe behaviour disorder with a mentally handicapped young woman in a community setting, in *Residential Care: A Reader in Current Theory and Practice* (eds R. Walton and D. Elliott), Pergamon, London, pp.139–148.

Mansell, J. (1988a) *Staffed Housing for People with Mental Handicaps: Achieving Widespread Dissemination*, South East Thames Regional Health Authority/Natiomnal Health Service Training Authority.

Mansell, J. (1988b) Training for service development, in *An Ordinary Life in Practice: Developing Comprehensive Community-Based Services for People with Learning Disabilities* (ed. D. Towell), King's Fund Centre, London, pp.129–140.

Mansell, J. (1989) Evaluation of training in the development of staffed housing for people with mental handicaps. *Mental Handicap Research*, **2**, 137–151.

Mansell, J. (1994) Specialized group homes for persons with severe or profound mental retardation and serious problem behaviour in England. *Research in Developmental Disabilities*, **15**, 371–388.

Mansell, J. (1995) Staffing and staff performance in services for people with severe or profound learning disability and serious challenging behaviour. *Journal of Intellectual Disability Research*, **39**(1), 3–14.

Mansell, J. and Beasley, F. (1990) Severe mental handicap and problem behaviour: Evaluating the transfer from institutions to community care, in *Key Issues in Mental Retardation Research* (ed. W.I. Fraser), Routledge, London, pp.405–413.

Mansell, J. and Beasley, F. (1993) Small staffed houses for people with a severe learning disability and challenging behaviour. *British Journal of Social Work*, **23**, 329–344.

Mansell, J., Felce, D., de Kock, U. and Jenkins, J. (1982) Increasing purposeful activity of severely and profoundly mentally handicapped adults. *Behaviour Research and Therapy*, **20**, 593–604.

Mansell, J., Felce, D., Jenkins, J. and de Kock, U. (1982) Increasing staff ratios in an activity with severely mentally handicapped people. *British Journal of Mental Subnormality*, **28**, 97–99.

Mansell, J., Felce, D., Jenkins, J. *et al.* (1987) *Developing Staffed Housing for People with Mental Handicaps*, Costello, Tunbridge Wells.

Mansell, J. and Hughes, H. (1990) *Consultation to Camberwell Health Authority Learning Difficulties Care Group: Evaluation Report*, Tizard Centre, University of Kent at Canterbury.

Mansell, J., Hughes, H. and McGill, P. (1993) Maintaining local residential placements, in *Severe Learning Disabilities and Challenging Behaviour: Designing High-Quality Services* (eds E. Emerson, P. McGill and J. Mansell), Chapman & Hall, London, pp.260–281.

Mansell, J., Jenkins, J., Felce, D. and de Kock, U. (1984) Measuring the activity of severely and profoundly mentally handicapped adults in ordinary housing. *Behaviour Research and Therapy*, **22**, 23–29.

Mansell, J., McGill, P. and Emerson, E. (1993) Conceptualising service provision, in *Severe Learning Disabilities and Challenging Behaviour: Designing High-Quality Services* (eds E. Emerson, P. McGill and J. Mansell), Chapman & Hall, London, pp.69–93.

Martin, J.P (1984) *Hospitals in Trouble*, Blackwell, Oxford.

Martinussen, W. (1988) *Solidaritetens Grenser*, Universitetsforlaget, Oslo.

McConkey, R., Walsh, P.N. and Conneally, S. (1993) Neighbours' reactions to community services: Contrasts before and after services open in their locality. *Mental Handicap Research*, **6**, 131–141.

McCormick, M., Balla, D. and Zigler, E. (1975) Resident-care practices in institutions for retarded persons: A cross-institutional, cross-cultural study. *American Journal of Mental Deficiency*, **80**, 1–17.

McGill, P. and Emerson, E. (1992) Normalisation and applied behaviour analysis: Values and technology in human services, in *Normalisation: A Reader for the 1990s* (eds H. Smith and H. Brown), Routledge, London, pp.60–83.

McGill, P., Emerson, E. and Mansell, J. (1994) Individually designed residential provision for people with seriously challenging behaviours, in *Severe Learning Disabilities and Challenging Behaviour: Designing High-Quality Services* (eds E. Emerson, P. McGill and J. Mansell), Chapman & Hall, London, pp.119–156.

McGill, P. and Toogood, S. (1993) Organizing community placements, in *Severe Learning Disabilities and Challenging Behaviour: Designing High-Quality Services* (eds E. Emerson, P. McGill and J. Mansell), Chapman & Hall, London, pp.232–259.

McKnight, J. (1987) Regenerating community. *Social Policy*, (Winter), 54–58.

Mercer, J. (1973) *Labeling the Mentally Retarded*, University of California Press, Berkeley, CA.

Meyer, R. (1980) Attitudes of parents of institutionalized mentally retarded individuals towards deinstitutionalization. *American Journal of Mental Deficiency*, **85**, 184–187.

Michels, R. (1962) *Political Parties*, The Free Press, New York.

Mittler, P.J. (1987) Staff development: Changing needs and service contexts in Britain, in *Staff Training in Mental Handicap* (eds J. Hogg and P.J. Mittler), Brookline Books, Cambridge, MA.

Moores, B. and Grant, G.W.B. (1976) On the nature and incidence of staff:patient interactions in hospitals for the mentally handicapped. *International Journal of Nursing Studies*, **13**, 69–81.

Moos, R.H. (1980) The environmental quality of residential care settings. *Environmental Design Research Association*, **11**, 7–21.

Morris, P. (1969) *Put Away: A Sociological Study of Institutions for the Mentally Retarded*, Routledge & Kegan Paul, London.

Murphy, G. (1993) Understanding challenging behaviour, in *Severe Learning Disabilities and Challenging Behaviours: Designing High Quality Services* (eds E. Emerson, P. McGill and J. Mansell), Chapman & Hall, London, pp.37–68.

Murphy, G. and Clare, I. (1991) MIETS: A service option for people with mild mental handicaps and challenging behaviour or psychiatric problems: 2 assessment treatment and outcome for service users and service effectiveness. *Mental Handicap Research*, **4**, 180–206.

Nakamura, R.T. (1987) The textbook process and implementation research. *Policy Studies Review*, **7**(1), 142–154.

National Health Service Management Executive (1992) *Health Services Guidance (92)42. Health Services for People with Learning Disabilities (Mental Handicap)*, National Health Service, London.

Nielsen, K.B. (1983) Fremtiden for en stor centralinstitution. *Psykisk Utvecklingshämning*, **85**(1), 16–22.

Nihira, K., Foster, R., Shellhaas, M. and Leland, H. (1974) *AAMD Adaptive Behavior Scale*, American Association on Mental Deficiency, Washington, DC.

Nirje, B. (1969) The principle of normalization and its human management implications, in *Changing Patterns in Residential Services for the Mentally Retarded* (eds R. Kugel and W. Wolfensberger), The President's Committee on Mental Retardation, Washington, DC, pp.179–195.

Nirje, B. (1992) *The Normalization Principle Papers*, Centre for Handicap Research, Uppsala.

North Western Regional Health Authority (1983) *A Model District Service*, North Western Regional Health Authority, Manchester.

NOU 1985:34 (Public committee report): *Levekår for psykisk utviklingshemmete*.

Novick, L.J. (1967) Easing the stress of moving day. *Hospitals*, **41**, 6–10.

Novak, A.R. and Berkely, T.R. (1984) A systems theory approach to deinstitutionalization policies and research, in *International Review of Research in Mental Retardation*, volume 12 (eds N. Ellis and N. Bray) Academic Press Inc., Orlando, FL.

O'Brien, J. (1987) A guide to life style planning: Using The Activities Catalogue to integrate services and natural support systems, in *The Activities Catalogue: An Alternative Curriculum for Youth and Adults with Severe Disabilities* (eds B.W. Wilcox and G.T. Bellamy) Paul H. Brookes Publishing Co., Baltimore, MD, pp.175–189.

O'Brien, J. and Lyle O'Brien, C. (1991) *More Than Just a New Address: Images of Organization for Supported Living Agencies*, Responsive Systems Associates, Lithonia, GA.

O'Brien, J. and Tyne, A. (1981) *The Principle of Normalisation: A Foundation for Effective Services*, Campaign for Mentally Handicapped People, London.

O'Neill, J., Brown, M., Gordon, W. and Schornborn, R. (1985) The impact of deinstitutionalization on activities and skills of severely/profoundly mentally retarded multiplyhandicapped adults. *Applied Research in Mental Retardation,* **6**, 361–371.

O'Toole, L.J. (1989) Goal multiplicity in the implementation setting: Subtle impacts and the case of wastewater treatment privatization. *Policy Studies Journal,* **18**(1), 1–20.

O'Toole, L.J. and Montjoy, R.S. (1984) Interorganizational policy implementation: A theoretical perspective. *Public Administration Review,* (November/December), 491–503.

Olsen, J.P. (1988) Statsstyre og reformforslag, in *Statsstyre og Institusjonsutforming* (ed. J.P. Olsen), Universitetsforlaget.

Orlowska, D., McGill, P. and Mansell, J. (1991) Staff–staff and staff–resident verbal interactions in a community-based group home for people with moderate and severe mental handicaps. *Mental Handicap Research,* **4**, 3–19.

Osborne, D. (1992) Governing in the 90s: How Governor Weld intends to reinvent state government. *Boston Globe,* January 2, 65 and 68–69.

Oswin M. (1978) *Children Living in Long-Stay Hospitals,* Heinemann, London.

Ot. prp. nr49 (1987–88) Midlertidig lov om avvikling av institusjoner og kontrakter om privatpleie under HVPU og lov om endringer i lov av 19 juni 1969 om sykehus m.v.

Ottenbacher, K.J. (1991) Statistical conclusion validity: An empirical analysis of multiplicity in mental retardation research. *American Journal on Mental Retardation,* **95**(42), 421–427.

Palmér, R. (1974) *Prediction of Work Performance and Work Adjustment in Mentally Retarded Adults,* Esselte Studium, Stockholm.

Parmenter, T. (1992) Quality of life of people with developmental disabilities, in *International Review of Research in Mental Retardation,* volume 18 (ed. N.W. Bray), Academic Press, New York, pp.247–287.

Perlt, B. (1990) Fra lighed til frihed. *PU-bladet,* **92**(4), 8–12.

Pfeffer, J. (1981) *Power in Organizations,* Pittman, Boston.

Porterfield, J., Blunden, R. and Blewitt, E. (1980) Improving environments for profoundly handicapped adults: Using prompts and social attention to maintain high group engagement. *Behavior Modification,* **4**, 225–241.

Powell, T.J. (1987) *Self-help Organizations and Professional Practice,* National Association of Social Workers, Silver Spring, MD.

Pratt, M.W., Bumstead, D.C. and Raynes, N.V. (1976) Attendant staff speech to the institutionalised retarded: Language use as a measure of the quality of care. *Journal of Child Psychology and Psychiatry,* **17**, 133–143.

President's Panel on Mental Retardation (1962) *A Proposed Program for National Action to Combat Mental Retardation,* U.S. Government Printing Office, Washington, DC.

Radford, J. and Tipper, A. (1988) *Starcross; Out of the Mainstream,* The Roehr Institute, Canada, p.82.

Rasmussen, M. (1972) De stora centralinstitutionernas framtid. *Psykisk Utvecklingshämning,* **74**(2), 16–19.

Rawlings, S. (1985) Behaviour and skills of severely retarded adults in hospitals and small residential homes. *British Journal of Psychiatry,* **146**, 358–366.

Raynes, N., Sumpton, R.C. and Flynn, M.C. (1987) *Homes for Mentally Handicapped*

People. Tavistock Publications, London.

Reid, D.H., Parsons, M.B. and Green, C.W. (1989) *Staff Management in Human Services: Behavioral Research and Application*, Charles C. Thomas, Springfield, IL.

Report of the Committee of Enquiry into Mental Handicap Nursing and Care (Chaired by P. Jay), (1979), Her Majesty's Stationery Office, London.

Report of the Committee of Inquiry into Allegations of Ill-treatment and other Irregularities at the Ely Hospital Cardiff (Cmnd 3975), (1969), Her Majesty's Stationery Office, London.

Report of the Committee of Inquiry at Farleigh Hospital (Cmnd 4557), (1971), Her Majesty's Stationery Office, London.

Report of the Committee of Inquiry on Normansfield Hospital (Cmnd 7537), (1978), Her Majesty's Stationery Office, London.

Report of the Committee of Inquiry into South Ockendon Hospital, (1974), Her Majesty's Stationery Office, London.

Report of the Committee of Inquiry into Whittingham Hospital (Cmnd 4861), (1972), Her Majesty's Stationery Office, London.

Report of the Joint Central and Local Government Working Party on Public Support for Residential Care (Chaired by J. Firth), (1987), Her Majesty's Stationery Office, London.

Report of the Royal Commission on the Law Relating to Mental Illness and Mental Deficiency (Chaired by Baron Percy), (Cmnd 169), (1957), Her Majesty's Stationery Office, London.

Repp, A.C., Barton, L.E. and Brulle, A.R. (1982) Naturalistic studies of mentally retarded persons V: The effects of staff instructions on student responding. *Applied Research in Mental Retardation*, **3**, 55–65.

Richardson, A. and Goodman, M. (1983) *Self-help and Social Care: Mutual Aid Organisations in Practice*, Policy Studies Institute, London.

Romer, D. and Heller, T. (1983) Social adaptation of mentally retarded adults in community settings: A social-ecological approach. *Applied Research in Mental Retardation*, **4**, 303–314.

Rotegard, L.L., Bruininks, R.H., Holman, J.G. and Lakin, K.C. (1985) Environmental aspects of deinstitutionalization, in *Living and Learning in the Least Restrictive Environment* (eds R.H. Bruininks and K.C. Lakin), Paul H. Brookes Publishing Co., Baltimore, MD, pp.141–152.

Rothman, D. (1971) *The Discovery of the Asylum: Social Order and Disorder in the New Republic*, Little, Brown & Co., Boston, MA.

Rothman, D. and Rothman, S.M. (1984) *The Willowbrook Wars*, Harper & Row, New York.

Rowbotham, S. (1973) *Woman's Consciousness, Man's World*, Penguin, Harmondsworth.

Saathoff, G.B., Cortina, J.A., Jacobson, R., Aldrich, C.K. (1992) Mortality among elderly patients discharged from a state hospital. *Hospital and Community Psychiatry*, **43**, 280–281.

Salomonsen, P. (1988) *Udflytning Af Psykisk Utviklingshaemmede*, Aalborg Universitetsforlag, Aalborg.

Saloviita, T. (1990) *Adaptive Behaviour of Institutionalized Mentally Retarded Persons*, Jyväskylä Studies in Education, Psychology and Social Research (Serial No. 73), University of Jyväskylä.

Saloviita, T. (1992) Back to community: a study on deinstitutionalization of persons with mental handicap. Tampere: The Finnish League of the Association for Persons with Developmental Disabilities (in Finnish).

Sandler, A. and Thurman, S.K. (1981) Status of community placement research: Effects on retarded citizens. *Education and Training of the Mentally Retarded*, **16**, 245–251.

Sandvin, J.T. (1992) Fra særomsorg til særlig omsorg, in *Fra Særomsorg Tilsærlig Omsorg* (ed. T. Visnes), Universitetsforlaget, pp.61–93.

Saxby, H., Thomas, M., Felce, D. and de Kock, U. (1986) The use of shops, cafés and public houses by severely and profoundly mentally handicapped adults, *British Journal of Mental Subnormality*, **32**(63), 69–81.

Schalock, R.H. (1989) *The Quality of Life Questionnaire*, personal communication, Hastings, Nebraska.

Schalock, R.L. (1990) *Quality of Life: Perspectives and Issues*, American Association on Mental Retardation, Washington, DC.

Schalock, R., Keith, K., Hoffman, K. and Karan, O. (1989) Quality of life: Its measurement and use. *Mental Retardation*, **27**, 25–31.

Schalock, R., and Lilley, M. (1986) Placement from community-based mental retardation programs: How well do clients do after 8 to 10 years? *American Journal of Mental Deficiency*, **90**, 669–676.

Scheerenberger, R.C. (1976) *Deinstitutionalization and Institutional Reform*, Charles C. Thomas, Springfield, IL.

Scheerenberger, R.C. (1981) Deinstitutionalization: Trends and difficulties, in *Deinstitutionalization and Community Adjustment of Mentally Retarded People, AAMD Monograph No.4.* (eds R.H. Bruininks *et al.*), American Association on Mental Deficiency, Washington, DC, pp.3–13.

Schmidt, H.B. (1985) Institutionskulturens sidste vers. *Psykisk Utvecklingshämning*, **87**(3), 22–26.

Schubert, M.A. and Borkman, T.J. (1991) An organizational typology of self-help groups. *American Journal of Community Psychology*, **19**, 769–788.

Schultz, T. (1984) Ekonomin vid utflyttning från anstalter. *Psykisk Utvecklingshämning*, **86**(4), 1–6.

Schulz, R. and Brenner, G. (1977) Relocation of the aged: A review and theoretical analysis. *Journal of Gerontology*, **32**, 323–333.

Scull, A. (1977) *Decarceration*, Polity Press, Cambridge, MA.

Scull, A. (1993) *The Most Solitary of Afflictions: Madness and Society in Britain*. The Bath Press, Avon.

Segal, R.M. (1969) The Association for Retarded Children: A Force for Social Change. Brandeis University, Waltham, MA. Dissertation.

Seligman, A. (1992) *The Idea of Civil Society*, The Free Press, New York.

Seltzer, G. (1980) Residential satisfaction and community adjustment. Paper presented at the *104th Annual Conference of the American Association on Mental Deficiency*, San Francisco, May.

Selznick, P. (1992) *The Moral Commonwealth: Social Theory and the Promise of Community*, University of California Press, Berkeley, CA.

Seys, D. and Duker, P. (1988) Effects of staff management on the quality of residential care for mentally retarded individuals. *American Journal on Mental Retardation*, **93**, 290–299.

Shea, J.R. (1992) From standards to compliance, to good services, to quality lives: Is this how it works? *Mental Retardation*, 30(3), 143–150.

Shearer, A. (1986) *Building Community: With People with Mental Handicaps, their Families and Friends*, King's Fund, London.

Shiell, A., Pettipher, C., Raynes, N. and Wright, K. (1992) The costs of community residential facilities for adults with a mental handicap in England. *Mental Handicap Research*, 5, 115–129.

Shiell, A., Pettipher, C., Raynes, N. and Wright, K. (1993) A cost-function analysis of residential services for adults with a learning disability. *Health Economics*, 2, 247–256.

Simon, H. (1945) *Administrative Behaviour*, The Free Press, New York.

Smith, G. (1990) *Supported Living: New Directions in Services to People with Developmental Disabilities*, NASMRPD, Alexandria, VA.

Smith, G. (1991) What's going on out there? Supported living and new directions. Paper presented at the Annual NARC Meeting, Minneapolis, Minnesota, in *Supported Living Monograph*, volume 1, National Association of Private Residential Resources, Arlington, VA.

Smull, M. (1989) *Crisis in the Community*, University of Maryland, Applied Research and Evaluation Unit, Baltimore, MD.

Smull, M. (1993) Sharing power and a system of supports. *Amercian Association on Mental Retardation News and Notes*, 6, 1–2.

Smull, M. and Bellamy, G.T. (1991) Community services for adults with disabilities, in *Critical Issues in the Lives of People with Severe Disabilities* (eds L.H. Meyer, C.A. Peck and L. Brown), Paul H. Brookes Publishing Co., Baltimore, MD, pp.527–536.

Socialstyrelsen (1987) Gruppbostäder – Aktuella frågeställningar kring utformning, personalutveckling och samverkan. Rapport. Stockholm: Socialstyrelsen.

Söder, M. (1978) Anstalter för utvecklingsstörda. En histiorisk-sociologisk beskrivning av utvecklingen, Stockholm: ALA.

Sonn, J. (1984) Institutionsavveckling genom utveckling. *Psykisk Utvecklingshämning*, 86(2), 9–13.

Sonnander, K. and Nilsson-Embro, A. (1984) *Utvecklingsstördas livskvalitet* (Quality of Life among the Mentally Retarded), Uppsala, Prosjekt Mental Retardation.

SOU 1946:24 Förslag till effektiviserad kurators- och arbetsförmedlingsverksamhet för partiellt arbetsföra m m.

Specht, D. and Nagy, M. (1986) *Social Supports Research Project: Report of Findings*, Western Massachusetts Training Consortium, Holyoke, MA.

St. meld. nr 67 1986–87: Ansvar for tiltak og tenester for psykisk utviklingshemma.

St. prp. 36 (1960–61) (Parliamentary Bill): Om videre utbygging av åndssvakeomsorgen.

Stanley, B. and Roy, A. (1988) Evaluating the quality of life of people with mental handicaps: A social validation study. *Mental Handicap Research*, 1, 197–210.

Stockholms läns landsting, (1977) Omsorgsvården i Stockholms län – mål och behov 1977–87. Stockholm: Omsorgsnämnden.

Sutter, P., Mayeda, T., Call, T. *et al.* (1980) Comparison of successful and unsuccessful community placed mentally retarded persons. *American Journal of Mental Deficiency*, 85, 262–267.

Taylor, H., Kagay, M. and Leichenko, S. (1986) The ICD Survey of Disabled

Americans Conducted by Louis Harris and Associates, New York: The International Center for the Disabled and Washington, DC: National Council for the Handicapped.

Taylor, S.J. (1988) Caught in the continuum: A critical analysis of the principles of the least restrictive environment. *Journal of the Association of Persons with Severe Handicaps*, **13**, 41–53.

Taylor, S.J. (1991) Toward individualized community living, in *Life in the Community*, volume 1 (eds S.Taylor, R. Bogdan and J.A. Racino), Paul H. Brookes Publishing Co., Baltimore, MD, pp.105–111.

Taylor, S.J., Biklen, D. and Knoll, J. (eds) (1987) *Community Integration for People with Severe Disabilities*, Teachers College Press, New York.

Taylor, S.J., Bogdan, R. and Racino, J.A. (eds) (1991) *Life in the Community*, volume 1, Paul H. Brookes Publishing Co., Baltimore, MD.

Thomas, M., Felce, D., de Kock, U. *et al.* (1986) The activity of staff and of severely and profoundly mentally handicapped adults in residential settings of different sizes. *British Journal of Mental Subnormality*, **32**(63), 82–92.

Thompson, F.J. (1984) Implementation of health policy: Politics and bureaucracy, in *Health Politics and Policy* (eds T.J. Litman and L.S. Robins), John Wiley & Sons, New York, pp.145–168.

Thorarinsson, T. (1987) Institutionsavveckling. PM. Anförande vid NFPU:s kongress i Uppsala.

Thorsell, M. (1989) Uppföljning efter utflyttning, unpublished manuscript.

Thorsteinsdóttir, A. and Björnsdottir, L. (1991) Nyt fra Island. *PU-bladet*, **93**(4), 27–30.

Thousand, J., Burchard, S. and Hasazi, J. (1986) Field-based determination of manager and staff competencies in small community residences. *Applied Research in Mental Retardation*, **7**, 263–283.

Titmuss, R. (1974) *Social Policy*, Allen & Unwin, London.

Tizard, J. (1960) Residential Care of Mentally Handicapped Children. *British Medical Journal*, 2 April, pp.1044.

Tizard, J. (1964) *Community Services for the Mentally Handicapped*, Oxford University Press, London.

Tønnies, F. (1912) *Gemeinschaft und Gesellschaft*, Berlin.

Toogood, A., Emerson, E., Hughes, H. *et al.* (1988) Challenging behaviour and community services: 3. Planning individualised services. *Mental Handicap*, **16**, 70–74.

Tøssebro, J. (1990a) *Spørreundersøkelsen velferd for psykisk utviklingshemmete: Gjennomføring og frekvensfordelinger*, Notat 6 i serien Fra Særomsorg til Næromsorg, THH/Allforsk/ISS, Trondheim.

Tøssebro. J. (1990b) *Spørreundersøkelsen 'Pårørendes syn på HVPU og HVPU-reformen'* – *Gjennomføring og frekvensfordeling*. Notat nr6 i serien 'Fra Særomsorg til Næromsorg', Trondheim, THH.

Tøssebro, J. (1991) Fra 'big is beautiful' til 'smått er godt'. Paper presented at *Sharing a Vision of the Future: Nordic Contributions Conference*, FUN, Uppsala, 3–4 September. (Revised version to appear in *American Journal on Mental Retardation*.)

Tøssebro, J. (1992a) Hvorfor så negative, in *Mot Normalt? Omsorgsideologier i forandring* (ed. J.T. Sandvin), Universitetsforlaget, pp.91–124.

Tøssebro, J. (1992b) *Institutsjonsliv i Velferdsstaten*, Ad Notam Gyldendal, Oslo.

Towell, D. (1988) (ed.) *An Ordinary Life in Practice: Developing Comprehensive*

Community-Based Services for People with Learning Disabilities, King's Fund, London.

Towell, D. and Beardshaw, V. (1991) *Enabling Community Integration: The Role of Public Authorities in Promoting an Ordinary Life for People with Learning Disabilities in the 1990s*, King's Fund, London.

Trojan, A., Halves, E., Wetendorf, H. and Bauer, R. (1990) Activity areas and developmental stages in self-help groups. *Nonprofit and Voluntary Sector Quarterly*, **19**, 263–278.

Turnbull, H.R. (1991) *The Communitarian Perspective: Thoughts on the Future for People with Developmental Disabilities*, Beach Center on Families and Disability, University of Kansas at Lawrence, Lawrence, KS.

Turnbull, H.R., Boggs, E., Brooks, P.O. and Biklen, D.P. (1981) *The Least Restrictive Alternative: Principles and Practices*, American Association on Mental Deficiency, Washington, DC.

Tuvesson, B. (1994) *Nära varandra igen*, Landstinget Skaraborg, Mariestad.

Tyne, A. (1978) Participation by families of mentally handicapped people in policy making and planning. Paper presented to the *Personal Social Services Council*, London.

Vitello, S. J., Atthowe, J. M. and Cadwell, J. (1983) Determinants of community placement of institutionalised mentally retarded persons. *American Journal of Mental Deficiency*, **87**, 539–545.

Walker, C., Ryan, T. and Walker, A. (1993) *Quality of Life After Resettlement for People with Learning Disabilities, Summary of the Report to the North West Regional Health Authority*, Department of Sociological Studies, Sheffield.

Webb, A.Y. (1988) *Closing Institutions: One State's Experience*, New York State Office of Mental Retardation and Developmental Disabilities, Albany, NY.

Weinstock, A., Wulkan, P., Colon, C.J. *et al.* (1979) Stress inoculation and interinstitutional transfer of mentally retarded individuals. *American Journal of Mental Deficiency*, **83**, 385–390.

Weiss, J.A. (1987) Pathways to cooperation among public agencies. *Journal of Policy Analysis and Management*, 7(1), pp.94–117.

Wells, L. and Macdonald, G. (1981) Interpersonal networks and postrelocation adjustment of the institutionalized elderly. *The Gerontologist*, **21**, 177–183.

Welsh Office (1978) *NIMROD: Report of a Joint Working Party on the Provision of a Community Based Mental Handicap Service in South Glamorgan*, Welsh Office, Cardiff.

Welsh Office (1983) *The All-Wales Strategy for the Development of Services for Mentally Handicapped People*, Welsh Office, Cardiff.

Welsh Office (1991) *The Review of the All-Wales Mental Handicap Strategy: Report on Consultancy on the Key Issues*, Welsh Office, Cardiff.

Welsh Office (1992) *The All-Wales Mental Handicap Strategy: Framework for Development from April 1993*, Welsh Office, Cardiff.

Whiffen, P. (1984) *Initiatives in In-service Training: Helping Staff to Care for Mentally Handicapped People in the Community*, Central Council for Education and Training in Social Work, London.

Willer, B. and Intagliata, J. (1984) An overview of the social policy of deinstitutionalization, in *International Review of Research in Mental Retardation*, volume 12 (eds N. Ellis and N. Bray), Academic Press Inc., Orlando, pp.1–23.

Wolfensberger, W. (1969) The origin and nature of our institutional models, in *Changing Patterns in Residential Services for the Mentally Retarded* (eds R. Kugel and W. Wolfensberger), President's Committee on Mental Retardation, Washington, DC, pp.59–171.

Wolfensberger, W. (1972) *Normalisation: The Principle of Normalisation in Human Services*, National Institute on Mental Retardation, Toronto.

Wolfensberger, W. (1975) *The Origin and Nature of our Institutional Models*, Human Policy Press, Syracuse, NY.

Wolfensberger, W. (1992) *A Brief Introduction to Social Role Valorization as a High–order Concept for Structuring Human Services*, 2nd edn, Syracuse University, Syracuse.

Wolfensberger, W. (1992) Deinstitutionalization policy: How it is made, by whom and why. *Clinical Psychology Forum*, **39**, 7–11.

Wolfensberger, W. and Glenn, L. (1975) *Program Analysis of Service Systems: A Method for the Quantitative Evaluation of Human Services*, National Institute of Mental Retardation, Toronto.

Wolfensberger, W. and Thomas, S. (1983) *PASSING: Programme Analysis of Service Systems' Implementation of Normalisation Goals*, National Institute on Mental Retardation, Toronto.

Wood, J.R.A. (1989) Comparing interactions in two hospital wards for people with mental handicaps: A pilot study. *Mental Handicap Research*, **2**, 3–17.

Woods, P. and Cullen, C. (1983) Determinants of staff behaviour in long-term care. *Behavioural Psychotherapy*, **11**, 4–17.

Wright, E.C., Abbas, K.A. and Meredith, C. (1974) A study of the interactions between nursing staff and profoundly retarded children. *British Journal of Mental Subnormality*, **20**(1), 38.

Wright, B., King, M.P. and NCSL Task Force on Developmental Disabilities (1991) *Americans with Developmental Disabilities: Policy Directions for the States*, CO: National Conference of State Legislatures, Washington, DC and Denver.

Zigler, E. and Balla, D. (1977) Impact of institutional experience on the behavior and development of retarded persons. *American Journal of Mental Deficiency*, **82**, 1–11.

Zigler, E., Balla, D. and Kossan, N. (1986) Effects of types of institutionalization on responsiveness social reinforcement, wariness and outer directedness among low-MA residents. *American Journal of Mental Deficiency*, **91**, 10–17.

Zigler, E., Hodapp, R. and Edison, M. (1990) From theory to practice in the care and education of mentally retarded individuals. *American Journal on Mental Retardation*, **95**, 1–12.

Zweig, J. and Csank, I. (1975) Effects of relocation on chronically ill geriatric patients of a medical unit: Mortality rates. *Journal of the American Geriatrics Society*, **23**, 132–136.

Index

Page numbers in **bold** refer to figures and page numbers in *italic* refer to tables.